NETTLE
POWER

FORAGE, FEAST & NOURISH YOURSELF
with This Remarkable Healing Plant

BRIGITTE MARS

Storey Publishing

The mission of Storey Publishing is to serve our customers by
publishing practical information that encourages
personal independence in harmony with the environment.

EDITED BY Carleen Madigan, Diana Rupp, and
  Sarah Guare Slattery
ART DIRECTION AND BOOK DESIGN BY
  Bredna Lago
TEXT PRODUCTION BY Jennifer Jepson Smith

COVER ILLUSTRATION BY Bredna Lago
  © Storey Publishing, front; © Gorba/
  Shutterstock.com, back t.; © Maisei Raman
  /Shutterstock.com, back b.
INTERIOR ILLUSTRATIONS BY © Katie
  Blanchard, vi, viii, 9, 11, 12, 22, 33, 36–37, 39,
  40, 43–44, 47–48, 50–51, 53–54, 59–60, 65, 71,
  74, 79, 85–86, 94, 112, 121, 129, 135
ADDITIONAL ILLUSTRATIONS BY © artform
  /Shutterstock.com, 15; © Gorba/Shutterstock
  .com, 14 t.; © Internet Archive Book
  Images/no restrictions/Wikimedia Commons,
  69; © Maisei Raman/Shutterstock.com, 14 b.;
  © Quagga Media/Alamy Stock Photo,
  3; Private Collection © Look and Learn
  /Bridgeman Images, 18; Richard Gaywood
  /Public domain/Wikimedia Commons, 16;
  William Shakespeare, Walter Crane/Public
  domain/Wikimedia Commons, 28
ALL OTHER GRAPHICS BY Bredna Lago
  © Storey Publishing

Text © 2024 by Brigitte Mars

The information in this book is true and
complete to the best of our knowledge. All
recommendations are made without guarantee
on the part of the author or Storey Publishing.
The author and publisher disclaim any liability
in connection with the use of this information.

The publisher is not responsible for web-
sites (or their content) that are not owned by
the publisher.

Storey books may be purchased in bulk for
business, educational, or promotional use.
Special editions or book excerpts can also be
created to specification. For details, please
contact your local bookseller or the Hachette
Book Group Special Markets Department at
special.markets@hbgusa.com.

Storey Publishing
210 MASS MoCA Way
North Adams, MA 01247
storey.com

Storey Publishing is an imprint of Workman
Publishing, a division of Hachette Book Group,
Inc., 1290 Avenue of the Americas, New York,
NY 10104. The Storey Publishing name and logo
are registered trademarks of Hachette Book
Group, Inc.

ISBNs: 978-1-63586-841-8 (paperback);
978-1-63586-842-5 (ebook)

Printed in Canada by Transcontinental Printing
on paper from responsible sources
10 9 8 7 6 5 4 3 2 1

Library of Congress Cataloging-in-Publication
  Data on file

DEDICATED TO
Sunflower Sparkle Mars,
Rainbeau Harmony Mars,
Jade Destiny Mars,
Solwyn Forest Stegall,
Luna Zara Mars,
Mitch Stegall,
and BethyLoveLight

CONTENTS

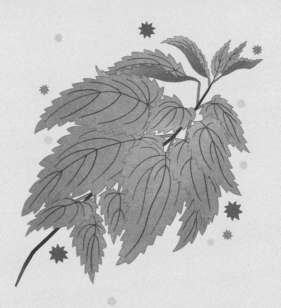

GREETINGS

Nettle has been one of my most valuable plant allies for several decades. My first experience with it was about 50 years ago, when an elderly German woman gave me a nettle plant from her homeland. I put it in my garden and forgot about it until two years later, when I was getting ready to move. I transplanted them (the single plant had multiplied to three) to a small, fenced area at our new home. Our family grew up and the nettles grew out. Soon there were 10,000 nettle plants growing between two buildings, without much sunlight or water other than unpredictable rain. I am amazed by nettle's vigor and resilience.

I also give thanks for the nourishment it offers. Many mornings during the growing season I harvest nettle tops to make a delicious, nutritious green juice. I toss the nettles in a blender with water and a few more ingredients, like a cut apple and half a lemon. In less than 2 minutes, I'm drinking a chlorophyll-rich elixir, infused with life force. That is freshness you can't buy at the store!

Over the past 40 years, I've shared countless recipes for providing nettle nourishment: nettle soup, nettle quiche, nettle popovers, nettle pesto, and so much more. Fresh nettle in season is bursting with vibrancy, but dried nettle is also wonderful. In late fall, I cut the nettles back and dry the leaves and stems in a paper bag, then use the dried plants to make nettle tea and soups to enjoy over the winter.

Each spring I start cuttings, so that I can share my love of nettles with friends, neighbors, and students. I take 5-inch cuttings from the tops of a hundred nettle plants, remove the bottom leaves, and place the stems in water until they grow little white roots. I put a jar of these rooted nettles on my porch and invite people to take them home to plant. I believe when I leave this planet, there will be thousands of nettle patches flourishing—all started by me!

For many years I have enjoyed the benefits of nettles and seen how many of my clients and students have improved their health by using this wonderful herb. At one time I had the beginnings of arthritis in two of my fingers, and I would avoid shaking hands with people to avoid the pain that it caused. After several sessions of being stung with nettles, I can no longer remember which fingers had the affliction.

When asked which herb to use, David Hoffmann, author of *Holistic Herbal*, has replied, "When in doubt, use nettles." I certainly agree that nettle is extraordinary as a healing and helpful plant.

I hope that the stories and recipes in this book help grow your love of nettle—and that you in turn spread the love to your own friends and neighbors. May nettle help heal your needs and infuse you with its light. Blessed be.

—Brigitte Mars

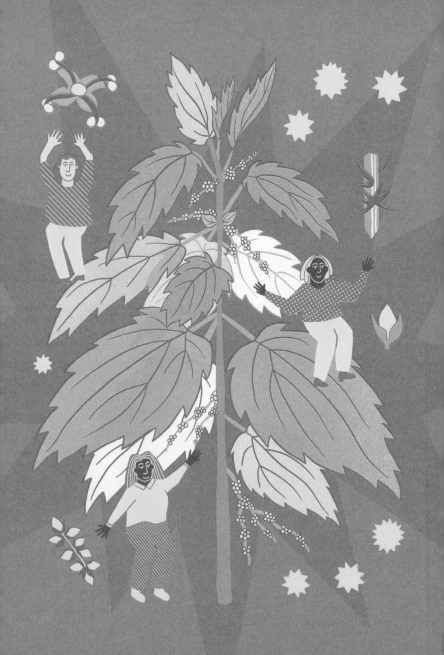

CHAPTER

1

THE VIRTUES OF NETTLE

Wouldn't you be delighted to know there is a wild plant that can help alleviate allergies; soothe arthritis; clear skin conditions; strengthen the kidneys; promote healthy bones, hair, and teeth; and be enjoyed as a delicious food, juice, or tea? Isn't it lovely that such a plant grows just about everywhere, from waste areas to gardens to grasslands to moist woods at various altitudes? The herb known as nettle is safe for young and old and has been used by millions of people for thousands of years to make medicine, textiles, rope, paper, dye, and more. Nettle is truly beautiful in its bounty.

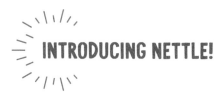

INTRODUCING NETTLE!

Nettle is one of the most remarkable plants on this planet. It is abundant, has a variety of uses, and offers many health-enhancing benefits. Because nettles grow so vigorously, many people consider the plant to be a weed. But as Ralph Waldo Emerson once said, "What is a weed? A plant whose virtues have not yet been discovered."

Herbs do not have to be rare, exotic, or covered with colorful flowers to be amazing and useful. Common as it is, nettle is nonetheless valued as a culinary, medicinal, cosmetic, and household herb. Nettle nourishes and strengthens the entire body. The Austrian philosopher, scientist, and artist Rudolf Steiner (1861–1925) called nettle "the heart of the world." Nettle radiates its healing force to the people and plants around it. And nettle's most distinctive feature—its sting—can be powerful medicine in itself, as we'll explore on page 11.

NETTLE'S RANGE AND APPEARANCE

Common nettle is originally native to Europe, Asia, and western North Africa, but it now grows on every continent except Antarctica, at elevations up to 9,000 feet. In the United States, it is found in every state except Hawaii, and there are other nettle species that are native to the Americas (see page 25).

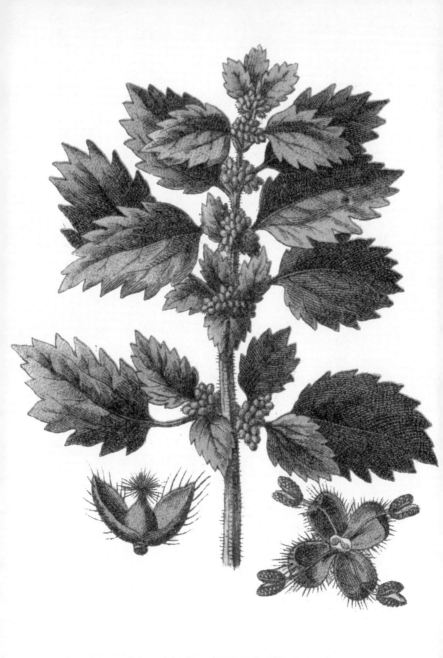

When the nettle is young, its leaf forms an excellent vegetable; when it matures, it has filaments and fibers like hemp and flax. Nettle fabric is as good as canvas. Chopped, the nettle is good for poultry; pounded it is good for cattle. The seed of the nettle mingled with fodder imparts a gloss to the coat of animals; its root mixed with salt produces a beautiful yellow color. It is besides excellent hay and can be cut twice. And what does the nettle require: Little earth, no attention, no cultivation. Only the seed falls as it ripens and is difficult to gather. That is all. With a little trouble, the nettle would be useful.

—VICTOR HUGO

Nettle grows wild where the land has been disturbed, usually near human habitation. It commonly grows in soft, easily compacted soil, often in large colonies in fens, hedgerows, grassland, moist woods, and waysides; along roadsides and garden fences; and near compost bins and other places where there is a lot of nitrogen, which it thrives on. Farmers recognize that land where nettles grow is rich enough for growing other crops. It also thrives in areas alongside running water where decomposing vegetation is washed downstream. In the garden, nettle spreads widely and quickly.

Botanical Origins

Nettle or common, greater, or European nettle, *Urtica dioica* (pronounced er-TI-kah die-OH-ee-kah), is a member of the Urticaceae (nettles) family. Some sources say the name "nettle" is derived from the Anglo-Saxon word *noedl*, meaning "needle," which may refer to nettle's use as a textile or fiber, as well as its sharp prickles. Others believe that nettle is from the Latin *nassa*, meaning "net," as its strong stems were woven into fishing nets and lines. The genus name *Urtica* is Latin for "I burn." The species name *dioica* means "two dwellings" or "two houses," in reference to nettle having either male or female flowers. *Urtica urens*, or small nettle, is smaller than the common nettle. It has shiny, rounded leaves and is an annual.

Nettle Nicknames

Nettle is known in English as stinging nettle, common nettle, big sting nettle, devil's leaf, devil's plaything, hoky-poky, hidgy-pidgy, Indian spinach, seven-minute itch, tanging nettle, and true nettle. *Urtica urens* is also known as lesser nettle and dog nettle.

A Nettle by Any Other Name

Around the world, the nettle is well known and is named:

Afrikaans:
brandnetel

Arabic:
nabat alqaras

Albanian:
hithër, hithra

Armenian:
yeghinj

Bengali:
nēṭala

Belarusian:
krapiva

Bulgarian:
kopriva

Bosnian:
kopriva

**Chinese
(Mandarin):**
xún má

Croatian:
kopriva

Czech:
kopřiva

Danish:
brændenælde

Dutch:
brandnetel

Esperanto:
urtiko

Estonian:
kõrvenõges

Finnish:
isonokkonen,
etelännokkonen

French: ortie
piquante

Filipino:
kulitis

Hawaiian:
ʻupena

German:
Brennnessel

Greek:
tsouknída

Hebrew:
sirpad

Hungarian:
csalán

Hindi:
bichchhoo bootee

Icelandic:
brenninetla

Indonesian:
jelatang

Italian:
ortica

Japanese:
irakusa

Javanese:
jelatang

Korean:
sswaegipul

Latin: urtica

Lithuanian:
dilgėlė

Mongolian:
khamkhuul

Norwegian:
brennesle

Persian:
gazaneh

Polish:
pokrzywa

Portuguese:
urtiga

Romanian:
urzica

Russian:
krapiva

Samoan:
u'u tui

Sanskrit:
bichu buti

Serbian:
kopriva

Slovak:
žihľava

Spanish:
ortiga

Sundanese:
jelatang

Swahili:
upupu

Swedish:
brännässla

Turkish:
ısırgan otu

Ukrainian:
kropyva

Welsh:
danadl poethion

Yiddish:
kropeve

Zulu:
izimbabazane,
sembabazane

Botanical Features

Nettle is an herbaceous perennial flowering plant, meaning it dies to the ground each winter but comes up again in spring. It's considered good looking, with its square stem, opposite leaves, and lovely, vibrant green color.

LEAVES, STALKS, AND STEMS

The coarsely toothed and veined leaves grow 2 to 5 inches long. Nettle plants have heart-shaped leaves at their base. The leaves are rough and oval-shaped with pointed tips. The leaves are darker on the top and paler underneath. The stems are hollow.

The foliage, leafstalks, and stems are all covered with thousands of tiny stiff, stinging, tubular prickles. Each sharp point is set in a swollen base, where cells collect the irritating fluid that is responsible for nettle's sting (see page 11). Where each leaf joins its main stem, you will usually find a pair of smaller leaves ready to branch out, should the plant be cut. The petiole or stalk that joins each leaf to the stem is somewhat long (2.5 inches), becoming shorter toward the top of the plant.

Nettle has erect branching stems that can grow to a height of 3 to 10 feet, although some annual varieties grow to only 10 to 12 inches. Plants growing near the coast and in open areas tend to be shorter. Stems can be processed into fibers that can be woven or made into paper.

FLOWERS

The green nettle flowers are minute and inconspicuous. They hang in long, branchlike clusters, often two from the axil of each leaf.

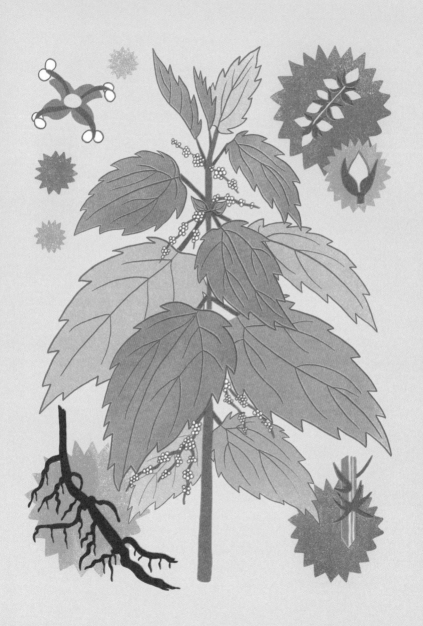

The male and female flowers appear on separate plants. The resulting "sexual dance of the nettles" can be beautiful to observe: The stamens of the male flower are curved in at the bud, but as they bloom, the stamens spring out to scatter their pollen. The female flower, which contains the stigmas and ovary, catches the pollen and ultimately produces a seed. This courtship can be observed on a sunny morning, usually from June to September, as male and female plants mingle their fertile portions. Herbalist Audrey Wynne Hatfield, author of *Pleasures of Wild Plants*, described it as "an enchanting early morning festival when the males gaily puff their pale golden pollen into the air to be caught by the females. And the plant fancier enthralled by novel plant habits will not be disappointed if he drags himself out of bed early enough to catch this graceful ritual."

FRUIT AND SEEDS

The oval fruit, a compressed polished nut, contains a single seed that is covered by the perianth, the outer part of the flower that is composed of the sepals and petals. The seeds are sticky and cling to clothing and the fur of passing animals—a useful way to find new homes for future plants. Seeds are also scattered by the wind and rain.

ROOTS

Nettle forms a circuit of horizontal underground stems called rhizomes. These roots are creeping, woody, and fibrous. If nettle stems are knocked down by animals or the rain and they touch the ground, fresh roots will descend from the stem and new plants will spring up.

THE INFAMOUS STING

Many people's first encounter with nettle is less than pleasant. If you unexpectedly brush up against the plant, you will get a painful sting and probably a rash. The sting is nature's way of protecting something valuable. Were it not for its sting, the plant would be devoured by wild animals.

Painful but Beneficial

Although many people are familiar with nettle's painful sting, most don't know that the sting offers hundreds of health benefits. As nutritionist and researcher Lelord Kordel wrote, "The sting of nettles is nothing compared to the pain that it heals." Nettle's sharp hairs, called trichomes, are hollow and act as hypodermic needles. A tiny amount of formic acid, acetylcholine, serotonin, and histamine held in the chamber at the base of the hair squirts into the skin. These compounds irritate the skin and create an antihistamine reaction, which ultimately reduces and clears out inflammation.

So how does the sting feel? It is intense for a few minutes, then over an hour or so mellows to a pleasant pins-and-needles kind of feeling, like a limb that has fallen asleep and is coming back to sensation. In some sensitive individuals, the stinging can last up to 12 hours, and in rare cases, 2 days or longer. After three or four successive sessions of exposure, the skin stops reacting. Then something curious happens: People experience some health *benefits*.

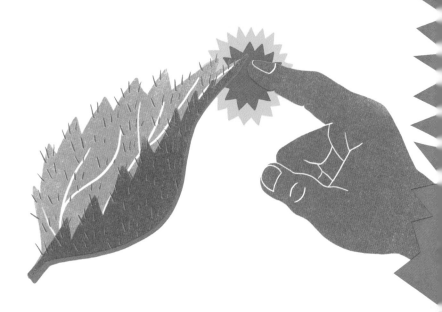

Relief from Inflammation

Thanks to a quick-acting process known as urtication that people have used to treat maladies for at least 2,000 years, exposure to nettle causes a rush of blood to the contacted area, which in turn produces a counterirritation and thereby reduces inflammation and gives temporary pain relief. Urtication stimulates energy to the nerves, muscles, capillaries, and lymphatics. Some people suggest that nettle offers pain relief partially because the immediate pain from the nettle sting causes one to ignore a deeper pain. In any case, nettle stings stimulate the body to secrete natural antihistamines. Urtication can help relieve the pain of arthritis, cold feet, gout, lumbago, muscular weakness, multiple sclerosis, neuritis, palsy, rheumatism, sciatica, and chronic tendonitis. In South America nettle urtication has been used to treat gangrene and thus avoid amputations.

The nineteenth-century herbalist and priest Father Sebastian Kneipp recommended nettles for relief from rheumatic pain when all other remedies had failed. He said, "The fear of the unaccustomed rod will soon give way to joy at its remarkable healing efficacy." In *King's American Dispensatory*, authors Harvey Wickes Felter, John King, and John Uri Lloyd reported that paralysis "is said to be cured by whipping the affected limbs" with fresh nettle leaves.

Nettle urtication is a valued treatment even today. Turn to page 76 for further information.

A Trick for Touching Nettles

When nettles are touched bravely, the tubes remain unbroken and do not sting, as the poet Aaron Hill wrote in his eighteenth-century poem "Verses Written on a Window in Scotland": "Tender-handed stroke a nettle, / And it stings you for your pains; / Grasp it like a man of mettle, / And it soft as silk remains."

Natural Remedies for Nettle's Sting

It is widely believed that wherever nettles grow, a remedy is close at hand. The juice of fresh nettle will cure the sting, as well as an application of the nettle root, chopped fine and applied as a poultice. Other herbs that can be used as a poultice are often found growing near the nettle plant, especially yellow dock (*Rumex crispus*). An old adage, quoted by Chaucer, is "Nettle in, Dock out. Dock rub Nettle out." A half teaspoon of yellow dock tincture can be mixed with 1 teaspoon baking

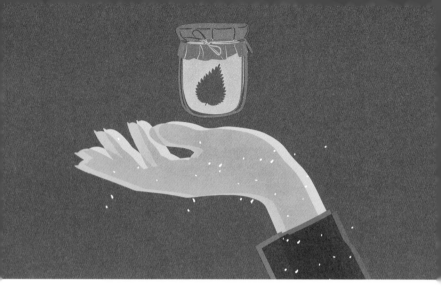

soda as a topical application for both nettle stings and ant
bites. Plantain (*Plantago major, P. lanceolota*) is another sooth-
ing antidote when used as a poultice. Jewelweed (*Impatiens
capensis, I. biflora*), rhubarb (*Rheum rhabarbarum*), peppermint (*Mentha × piperita*), sage (*Salvia officinalis*), mullein
(*Verbascum thapsus*), or rosemary (*Rosmarinus officinalis*) may
also be useful as a poultice. The rusty covering of young fiddle-
head ferns can also be rubbed onto nettle sting, as is done by
the Inuit people.

Making It Safe to Eat

None of the recipes included in this book will sting your mouth.
When nettles are heated, such as by boiling or steaming, the
formic acid quickly dissipates. Puréeing or juicing also breaks
up the tiny stinging hairs; once they're flattened, the formic acid
can no longer penetrate the body in a way that causes a stinging
sensation. Drying the plant will also remove its ability to sting.

THE HISTORY OF NETTLE

Throughout history, people have known which local plants provide food, medicine, or clothing. This knowledge was imperative to survival. Remains of nettle have been observed in deposits from three ice ages. Cremated bones in a Danish burial site from the later part of the Bronze Age (3000–1200 BCE) were wrapped in nettle cloth. Ancient burial sites unearthed in the western Chinese steppes revealed 2,000-year-old perfectly preserved nettle burial cloths. The Buddhist master Milarepa (1052–1135 CE) is said to have eaten only nettles for several years, so that his skin took on a greenish hue. He eventually developed legendary physical and psychic abilities.

More Historical Facts

In ancient Egypt, nettle seed oil was used as lamp fuel. Nettle was one of the important herbs in the European Wise Woman tradition.

Nettle is mentioned in the Bible in Job 30:7, Proverbs 24:31, Isaiah 34:13, Hosea 9:6, and Zephaniah 2:9.

Around the third century BCE, Hippocrates recommended nettle juice as a topical application for snake and scorpion bites as well as an antidote for poisoning from henbane and hemlock.

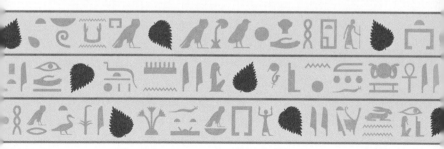

Ancient Roman soldiers spread some species of nettles into northern Europe, including *Urtica pilulifera*, which they whacked themselves with to increase circulation and keep warm. They also preserved nettles in salt and oil and applied the mixture as a rub to keep out the cold. A Latin inscription dating to the Roman occupation of Britain reads: "Take nettles and seethe them in oil, smear and rub all thy body therewith; the cold will depart away."

In Britain's old Wessex dialect, nettle was known as "wergulu." During the tenth century, nettle was one of nine sacred Celtic herbs along with chamomile, chervil, crab apple, fennel, mugwort, plantain, watercress, and either cockspur grass or wood betony (scholarly opinion about the identity of the ninth herb differs). Saint Patrick blessed nettle for its service to humans and animals. The Renaissance artist Albrecht Dürer (1471–1528) painted an angel flying heavenward with a stinging nettle in hand. Nicholas Culpeper, the great seventeenth-century British herbalist, recommended nettle against poisons and as a remedy against deadly nightshade and mandrake, as well as a treatment for dog bites.

Some settlers in seventeenth-century New England found that nettles followed them from England via imported cattle. They welcomed and documented it in a list of plants that grew of their own accord. The first record of nettle seeds being carried on purpose from England to New England dates from 1638, when a gardener named John Josselyn transported seed to the New World in tribute to their importance in the mother country.

Native American Uses

Native American people widely used nettles long before the arrival of Europeans, including the Cahuilla, Cherokee, Cree, Hesquiaht, Iroquois, Lakota, Paiute, Chippewa, Shoshone, Miwok, Pomo, Nuwa (Kawaiisu), Coast Salish, Skagit, Winnebago, Menominee, and Omaha nations. The Iroquois and Mohegans ate the greens as a vegetable, and the Ojibwe used nettles to treat urinary problems as well as dysentery. Native American women consumed nettle tea during pregnancy to strengthen the fetus, promote easy birth, and prevent hemorrhage during childbirth. Several Nevada nations burned nettle leaves in sweat lodges as an offering and to treat respiratory infections. The Nuwa (Kawaiisu) believed that if one desired a powerful dream, they should walk barefoot through a nettle patch to prepare themselves for entering the dream world. First Peoples of the Pacific Northwest stung themselves with nettles so they could stay awake on long whaling trips. Many nations—including the Winnebago, Coast Salish, Cupeño, Menominee, Omaha, and peoples of subarctic regions—wove nettle into robes, undershirts, cloaks, and ponchos.

NETTLE IN FOLKLORE

Legend and lore are steeped in references to nettle. Here are a few from various cultures and periods throughout the ages.

☆ In *The Wild Swans* by Hans Christian Andersen (1805–1875), a princess had to break the spell that had turned her 11 brothers into swans by weaving them each a cloak of nettles.

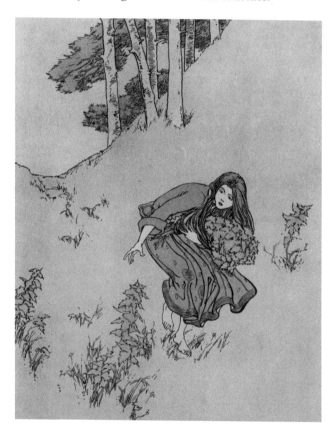

- ☼ In alchemy, nettle is under the dominion of the planet Mars, which governs plants with thorns or prickles (since Mars is the god of war) and the sign of Aries. It is also under the influence of Saturn.

- ☼ Nettle has long been scattered around the home or carried on one's person with yarrow (*Achillea millefolium*) to offer protection from danger.

- ☼ According to the Anglo-Saxon "Nine Herbs Charm" recorded in the tenth century, nettle was used as protection against "elf-shot," or unexplainable pains in humans or animals caused by the arrows of the elf folk.

- ☼ In Norse myth, nettles are associated with Thor, the god of thunder, and with Loki, the trickster god, whose magical fishing net is made from nettles.

- ☼ Celtic lore says that nettles indicate the presence of fairy dwellings nearby. The sting of the nettle is believed to offer protection against fairy mischief or dark magic.

- ☼ An Algonquian myth states that the Creator provided the inspiration for weaving nettle nets through the example of spiders spinning their webs.

- ☼ During thunderstorms, Tyroleans of Austria would throw nettles into the fire to protect their homes from being struck by lightning.

- ☼ In France, holding a bunch of nettles with yarrow would assuage fear in times of danger, and blowing through a hole in a nettle leaf was believed to improve poor vision, although the person blowing had to be "a woman who had never met her father."

☼ In Ireland, the last day of April was known as Nettlemas night. Boys would roam the streets after dark, carrying nettle bunches and stinging each other.

☼ When worn as an amulet, nettle was believed to give protection from negative influence. During the Middle Ages, a nettle patch was said to indicate the dwellings of elves and fairies and to give protection against sorcery.

☼ In England, nettle was used to drive the devil away.

☼ Nettle was believed to keep house trolls from spoiling the milk in Scandinavia.

☼ According to many European traditions, sprinkling nettle around a home was said to keep away any evil, and a pot of freshly cut nettles placed under a person's sickbed was said to speed their recovery.

☼ In European folklore, uttering a person's name as you pulled the plant out by its roots was used to cure fever.

☼ In Europe, herbs that grow in cemeteries, such as nettles, were said to be good for treating edema.

☼ In the language of flowers, if someone gives you a bouquet of nettle, they are trying to tell you they think you are cruel and spiteful.

☼ Nettle is the birthday plant of October 31 (Halloween).

☼ North American Indigenous folklore associates nettle with the trickster coyote and thus is a reminder to humankind of their foolishness in considering nettle a weed.

THE DOCTRINE OF SIGNATURES

The doctrine of signatures is an ancient belief system that a plant's appearance hints at what part of the body it can treat. The concept evolved from bits of astrology, alchemy, fact, and fantasy. The doctrine is founded on the belief that by observing a plant—the color of its flower, the shape of its leaf or root—you can determine its place in nature's plan. For example, nettle stems are strong and difficult to break, indicating the plant supports strength and structure in the body. Nettle is covered with hairs that sting, itch, and burn the skin when touched, suggesting it is a remedy to treat burns, rash, skin ailments, and itch as well as conditions that feel like "pins and needles," such as arthritis.

Its hairy appearance may have been what gave people the idea that nettles would improve hair growth. Nettle plants develop crystalline structures called cystoliths, suggesting that the plant helps wash away kidney stones (uric acid crystals).

Considering the fact that nettles grow abundantly and close to human population, part of their message might be "Use me lots!"

CHAPTER

2

GROWING, HARVESTING, AND FORAGING

By now we've learned that nettle is useful as medicine, food, and cosmetics and that even the sting has a purpose. (And those of us who have collected nettles for years don't mind the sting, knowing all the benefits this herb gives.) Since the value of the plant is undisputed, how can we obtain more of this beneficial botanical? The answer is simple: Grow, harvest, and even forage your own.

GROWING NETTLES

New plants can be grown from seeds, planted shallowly in early spring, or from a root division. The seeds take 10 to 14 days to germinate. Dividing a plant by the roots is best done in early spring, April and May. Like most perennials, new nettle plants are slow to get started but spread rapidly once established (usually by the third year).

In summer the seeds and plants can be harvested. In fall, at the end of the growing season, cut the plants back close to the ground. In winter nettle plants have no special requirements as they are hardy, die down, and lie dormant. If you're feeling intrepid, you can dig up some roots in autumn, place them in a growing tub, cover them with soil, and store them in an area protected from freezing (such as a cellar), where they will produce blanched, tender shoots that you'll appreciate in winter when few fresh garden vegetables are available.

Nettle does fine in cold climates, thriving in USDA Zones 3 to 10. Its ideal pH level is between 5.0 and 8.0. Nettles rarely get infested or diseased.

Where should you place nettle in the garden? It is kind to plant nettles out of reach of those who walk down your garden path, as the stinging experience is usually unpleasant for those who do not understand its benefits. Most people will also not want nettle to spread and may choose to plant them in containers.

Nettle Species

There are some 50 species of nettle, most of which grow in the tropics. Native to Eurasia, *Urtica dioica* has naturalized in north temperate and south temperate zones, including most of the United States, Canada, southern South America and the Andes, Asia, the Arctic, South Africa, and southern Australia. It's the most common form of nettle found in North America, along with *U. urens*, and the kind you're most likely to grow in your garden. With the exception of *U. ferox* (see below), all *Urtica* species are edible and can be used in the same way as *U. dioica*. Other plants that are known as nettles and in the Urtica family include:

U. californica. Grows on the California coast. Now classified as *U. gracilis* subsp. *gracilis*.

U. canadensis. Known as Canada nettle, Indian hemp. Now classified as *Laportea canadensis*.

U. cannabina. A Siberian species grown for its fiber content.

U. capitata. Known as common nettle. Now classified as *Boehmeria cylindrica*.

U. chamaedryoides. Known as southern nettle.

U. crenulata. Native to India, also grows in the United States. Has a very intense sting. Now classified as *Dendrocnide sinuata*.

U. dubia. Known as the European large-leafed nettle. Now classified as *U. membranacea*.

U. ferox. Grows in New Zealand. Its sting is very strong, and the plant is considered inedible.

U. gracilenta. Grows in the southern portion of the Rocky Mountains.

U. gracilis. Known as slim nettle, it's native to North America and has slender lance-shaped leaves and fewer stinging hairs than *U. dioica*.

U. heterophylla. Native to India, with a powerful sting. Now classified as *Girardinia diversifolia* subsp. *diversifolia*.

U. holosericea. Grows in the California desert and north to Washington, also in Australia.

U. hyperborea. Grows in India.

U. incisa. Grows in Australia.

U. lobulata. Grows in South Africa.

U. lyallii. *Grows* on the California coast and in the Pacific Northwest.

U. massaica. From tropical Africa.

U. parviflora. Grows in India. Now classified as *U. ardens*.

U. pilulifera. Native to the southern Europe/Mediterranean region, grows in India and South Africa. Species name means "pill-bearing nettle." Thought to have been brought to England by the Romans.

U. procera. Grows in the Rocky Mountains, a variety of *U. dioica*. Has male and female flowers on the same plant.

U. pumila. Grows in Eurasia and North America. Known as coolweed, richweed, stingless nettle, clearweed. Now classified as *Pilea pumila*.

U. purpurascens. Grows in the United States. Now classified as *U. chamaedryoides* subsp. *chamaedryoides*.

U. serra. Grows in wet areas of California, Oregon, and Washington between 5,000 and 10,000 feet. Now classified as *U. gracilis* subsp. *aquatica*.

U. stimulans. Known as the East Indian nettle; grows in India and the United States. Very powerful sting. Now classified as *Dendrocnide stimulans*.

U. thunbergiana. Native to Japan.

U. tuberosa. Grows in India. Features edible tubers. Now classified as *Pouzolzia zeylanica* var. *zeylanica*.

U. urens. Known as dwarf stinging nettle or dwarf nettle, this naturalized European plant grows in the United States, Australia, and South Africa. Grows to less than a foot tall and less hairy than *U. dioica*, with thin oval leaves. Annual rather than perennial plant.

U. urentissima. Known as devil's stinging nettle or dwarf stinger, it produces a sting that is said to last a year. From Java. Grows in India and the United States. Now classified as *U. spatulata*.

U. viridis. Grows in the Rocky Mountains. Narrow-leafed.

Laportea canadensis. Known as wood nettle. Similar to *U. dioica* but has terminal flower clusters, alternate leaves, and fewer stinging hairs. Edible and medicinal, like other nettles.

Some *Urtica* species do not have stinging hairs. Dead nettle and white nettle or blind nettle (*Lamium album,* also known as stingless nettle) are not related to *Urtica* species but are members of the mint family.

"The strawberry grows underneath the nettle,
And wholesome berries thrive and ripen best
Neighboured by   fruit of baser   quality"

Henry V.,
Act 1., Sc. 1

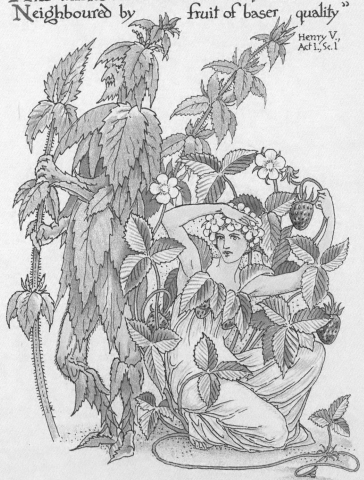

The Gardener's Friend

Not only does nettle have many medicinal and culinary uses, it also makes magic in the garden in distinctive ways.

Repels pests and diseases. Nettles can be made into a tea, cooled, and put in a spray bottle to make a natural pest repellent for plants. Simply boil the leaves and roots in water for half an hour, then strain and apply to afflicted plants to get rid of aphids, flea beetles, and plant lice, and to control mildew.

Similarly, there is a belief among British gardeners that the place where nettle is growing wild is the best place to plant an orchard. When nettles grow close to tomato plants, the tomatoes benefit from the formic acid, which protects the tomato against disease and is said to improve the flavor of the fruit.

Increases plant quality and seed production. Franz Lippert, an anthroposophist and leader in the biodynamic movement, observed that when nettles were grown close to peppers, tomatoes, potatoes, mustard, and coriander, those plants had at least a 30% increase in seed production. Root vegetables grown near nettles produced quality roots and were more disease resistant. Potatoes, parsley, and strawberries benefit from growing near nettles.

Boosts herbal essential oil content. Growing nettles near garden herbs increases the herbs' valuable essential oil content and thus their flavor and aroma, especially angelica (80%), valerian (20%), marjoram (10–20%), peppermint (10%), and sage (10%). Nettles planted next to angelica also help control blackfly infestation. Other companion plants that thrive near nettles in the wild include cow parsnip, horsetail, mint, and cleavers.

Fertilizes. Watering plants with nettle tea stimulates their growth and makes them more resistant to insect pests. It can also be used to water plants being transplanted. To make a nitrogen fertilizer, fill a bucket of nettles with water to cover and let soak for 6 to 10 days, then strain out the solids, dilute the liquid with 10 times the amount of water, and use as a fertilizer to water your garden. To create nettle fertilizer on a larger scale, pack a large nonmetallic container with fresh nettle plants and let the vessel fill with rainwater. Allow the mixture to steep and ferment for two weeks in warm weather or three weeks in cooler temperatures. Strain out and compost the solids. Dilute at a rate of 1 part fertilizer to 10 parts water and use to water garden vegetables like tomatoes.

Accelerates composting. When added to the compost pile, nettle hastens the breakdown process. Nettle has a carbon-to-nitrogen ratio comparable to barnyard manure, which encourages the decay of organic matter. Add to the compost either a nettle tea or the plant itself before it goes to seed.

Too Many Nettles?
Digging up the rhizomes is one way to control them. Use a digging fork to loosen the surrounding soil, pull up as much of the tangled roots as possible, spread them in a sunny place to dry completely, then compost. If nettles are cut down below the soil line three times for 3 years in a row, the plants will die.

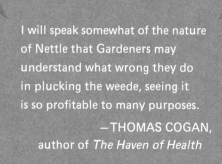

I will speak somewhat of the nature
of Nettle that Gardeners may
understand what wrong they do
in plucking the weede, seeing it
is so profitable to many purposes.

—THOMAS COGAN,
author of *The Haven of Health*

HARVESTING NETTLES

If all you need are the leaves and flowers, take only some tops from the plants; this promotes new growth. You might also thin plants growing together, as you would thin plants in your garden, to give the other plants more room. If you're collecting roots, which will destroy the plants, plant ripe seeds in the holes you've dug and fill the holes with soil.

Leaves are best taken just as the plant begins to flower, as the plants will still be directing energy to the leaves. Gather on a sunny morning, after the dew has risen and before the sun is hot. If possible, spray or water plants the day before you harvest them to clean off any dirt or debris. Leaves and flowers are usually harvested during the time of the full moon.

Roots generally are harvested in fall, after the plant has completed its cycle and the life force of the plant goes back into its roots and inner bark. Roots are said to be best when collected during the time of the new moon.

Leaves and Stems

Unless you wish to feel the burn, wear gloves, preferably made from leather, and protective clothing such as long sleeves, jeans, and closed-toe shoes. (If any mullein plants grow nearby, you can use them as makeshift potholders to protect your hands.) Stinging is less likely to occur when you pick the leaves from their underside, folding the top of the leaf inward. Note that the stinging may be more intense if you brush across the plant, rather than press into it.

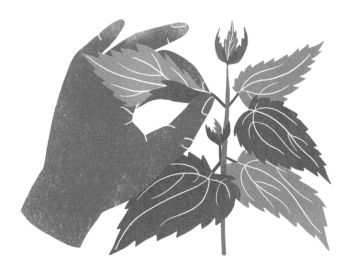

Using kitchen shears, cut the plant to about 3 inches above the root, or collect the top 10 inches. Be careful not to collect diseased or bug-infested parts. Thick paper bags are good for placing the collected plants into.

Collect tender shoots when they are less than 8 inches tall, ideally before the flowers form or when the upper leaves are still a pale green. Young plants will sometimes have a reddish or purplish tint, which is fine and natural. By cutting nettle tops throughout the growing season, you'll encourage the growth of fresh young green tips into fall. If the plants have grown taller than 8 inches and have not flowered yet, they can still be harvested for tea. Once the nettles have grown to about 12 inches, harvest only the very top two pairs of leaves, as the plant will have become too fibrous for making tea. Note, too, that after flowering, nettle develops cystoliths—tiny gritty particles of calcium carbonate—that can irritate the urinary tract if ingested in large quantities.

Seeds

Nettle seeds are used topically and internally as an anti-inflammatory agent that benefits the skin, hair, and nails. Nettle seed detoxifies both the liver and kidneys and improves their ability to cleanse the blood. Because of this, it is an antidote to poisonous plants and is also useful in cases of bee stings as well as spider, dog, and snake bites. It can also treat erectile dysfunction, goiter, and hypothyroidism and help prevent hair loss. A suggested dose as a thyroid tonic is 1 to 2 tablespoons daily.

Nettle seeds are best collected from midsummer to midautumn after the plant has flowered, although this depends on how hot summer is and how early winter comes. Pick when the seeds are fully dry, but still green and healthy looking.

To harvest, wear gloves and protective clothing (unless you have grown accustomed to the sting, or consider it therapeutic, as I do). Cut the fruiting tops of the plant, bundle them, and hang them to dry. Place some clean paper or piece of cloth underneath to catch the seeds as they fall. When totally dry, store the seeds in a glass jar and grind fresh as needed for seasoning. Or plant some seeds in your garden or a friend's.

Roots

The roots can be collected in fall. Using a shovel, dig in a circle 6 inches from the plant, loosening the dirt and gently pulling up the roots (rhizomes). Leave a third of the roots so the plant can regrow. Replace the earth and collect the roots in a bucket. Wash, then tincture when fresh, or dry for use as tea, tincture, capsule, or dye. (See Chapter 4 for recipes).

Gathering Guidelines for Foraging and Wildcrafting

Learning to grow or collect many different wild plants from your area will greatly enhance your connection to the earth. Save time, money, gas, the bees, your health, and the planet's health! Here are a few general tips for gathering plants safely and respectfully.

Carefully identify all plants. The most important rule of wildcrafting is to make sure you collect the proper species. Be sure you haven't collected any unwanted plants, and identify and leave behind any known endangered species. Use a good guidebook to identify plants.

Gather safely. Avoid collecting plants within 50 feet of a busy road, in areas that are sprayed with herbicides or pesticides, or in areas known to be polluted or contaminated.

Be respectful and joyful. Ask permission before gathering on private land. Ask permission from the herbs you gather, and give thanks.

Never take more than 10 percent of what's there and vary the places you collect from. Leave some plants for other aspiring herbalists! Collect plants when they are in their prime, not fading.

Harvest with the future in mind. For example, if all you need are the leaves and stems, take only some tops. By collecting nettle tops regularly, new growth will continue, which will allow you to harvest fresh young nettle tops over and over again.

Identify the grandfather or grandmother plant (the tallest, largest, first to bloom) and leave it in place to ensure the continuation of the strongest of the species.

Forage conservatively and harvest from the outside edges of the stand. Also help "thin" plants growing too closely together so that the other plants have more room. Cover holes after digging roots, and replant some of the ripe seeds, if available.

PRESERVING NETTLES

There are several ways to preserve harvested nettles, the most common being drying, as it is free, effective, and easy.

Drying

If you won't be using fresh nettles immediately, drying is the best method of preserving them so that their nutritional and therapeutic benefits can be enjoyed through the cold winter months until more plants are available the next spring. As a bonus, dehydrated herbs require only one-sixth the storage space of the fresh plant material.

I do not recommend washing nettle leaves and stems before drying because any droplets of water on the plant can lead to mold or dark spots. If you prefer to rinse the plants, swish them in a bowl or sink filled with cold water. Drain and then pat dry thoroughly with paper towels. (Alternatively, spin-dry using a salad spinner.) You can also try harvesting the day after a rain for naturally clean plants.

To dry the roots, scrub them well and cut large ones in half lengthwise to ensure quicker drying.

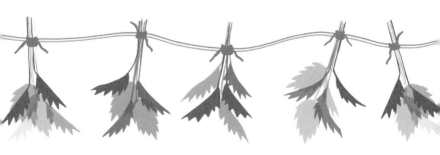

METHODS

There are a variety of ways to dry nettle. I encourage you to try the different methods listed here to see what works best for you. Air-drying usually takes a few days, while a dehydrator takes less than a day.

Paper bag method. My favorite way to dry nettle is to cut the top 10 inches or so off the plant using scissors and allow the tops to fall into a paper bag. Put the bag in a warm, dry place and give it a gentle shake daily until the nettles are fully dried. Drying herbs in a paper bag in the backseat of the car can be very effective.

Hanging. Tie 6 to 10 stems into a bunch with string and hang in a warm, dry, well-ventilated place away from direct sunlight. Be sure to allow adequate room between bunches for good air circulation.

Drying rack or screen. Spread leaves and stems in a single layer on a nylon, stainless steel, or fiberglass screen or in a shallow box and turn them several times a day to prevent mold. Setting up a fan nearby can ensure good airflow and speed up the process.

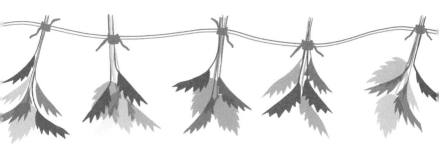

Alternatively, for herbs that contain a lot of moisture, I sometimes spread a clean sheet on the top floor (the hottest area of our home) and spread the herbs out on the sheet until they are dry.

Dehydrating. Set a dehydrator on its lowest temperature, usually the "herb" setting or 95 to 115°F (35 to 46°C). Remove the leaves from the stems or lay the cut tops in a single layer on the dehydrator trays. Use the upper shelves for moister leaves. Set to dry for 12 to 18 hours. (Note that it will take less time to dry the leaves than stems.)

STORING DRIED NETTLE

Given the right conditions, most leaves, stems, and roots will dry in 4 to 7 days. The leaves should crumble easily, and the stems should snap; if they bend and remain flexible, they probably contain moisture. To test a root for dryness, slice into it in a couple of places; if the center is dry to the touch, it's likely ready to be stored. Another method to test for dryness is to seal a sample of herb in a small, dry glass jar. If droplets of moisture appear on the lid, the plant needs to be dried more.

Make sure the nettle is fully dry before storing; otherwise it may develop mold. Clean, dry glass jars are the best for storing dried herbs for maximum shelf life. Pack the herbs into glass jars with lids and label them with the contents and the date. (A few months later you might not remember if it is a tea, spice, or remedy. With nettle, it could be all three!) Store the jars away from heat and light and use within 18 months.

Freezing

Freezing nettle is an easy way to add the plant's health benefits to dishes all year round. Rinse the nettles, place in a heatproof bowl, and cover with boiling water. Let stand for 5 minutes. Drain and then pack into freezer bags, squeezing out as much air as possible. Nettle keeps for up to 9 months in the freezer.

Canning

Canned nettles can be used in recipes of your choice after draining any excess water, or you can warm and eat them as a side dish. To prepare them, rinse the nettle, chop, and simmer in water until wilted. Pack into clean canning jars, leaving ½ inch of headspace. Add ½ teaspoon salt to each pint jar and 1 teaspoon salt to each quart. Cover the nettles and salt with boiling water, again leaving ½ inch of headspace. Screw on the lids. Process in a pressure cooker with boiling water at 10 pounds pressure, pints for 70 minutes and quarts for 90 minutes. Make sure the seals are tight when cooled.

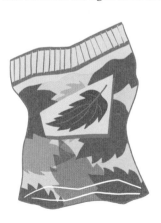
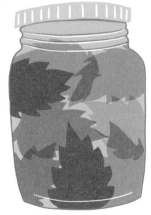

Nettles as Food Preservative

When dried nettles are placed among stored winter fruits, the fruits preserve longer, are more resistant to mold, and maintain their flavor better. Dried nettle can also be wrapped around apples, pears, root vegetables, and moist cheeses to deter pests and thus aid in their preservation. In years past, country villagers laid nettle leaves under cream cheese as a preservative.

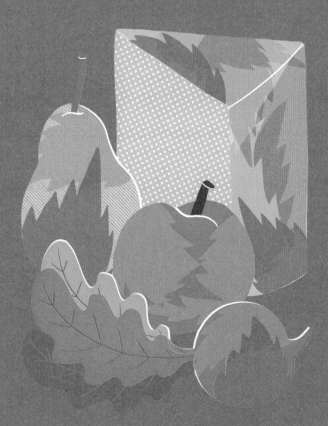

NETTLE TEXTILES AND PAPER

In addition to nettle's use as food and medicine, its stems can also be processed to yield fibers that are spun and woven into textiles. Nettle linen is of excellent quality and durability. The dried stalks are soaked in water, the outer skin is removed, and the inner fibers are carded or prepared for spinning into thread or yarn. Nettle fabric is still available to this day, especially in Europe and Asia, and is rather expensive. Another plant in the Urticaceae family, ramie (*Boehmeria nivea*), native to Asia, is today a major fiber plant.

Historically, nettle was also used to make paper in France and Siberia. Making nettle paper today is popular with scouts, foragers, and naturalists. Perhaps nettle paper will be made commercially again.

A History of Using Nettle for Cloth

Nettle provided cloth for northern Europeans long before hemp and flax were brought from the south. Nettle fibers were spun, coarsely or finely, into thread and used to make stout ropes, smooth fishing nets, sailcloth, canvas, fine linen, fine lace, and paper.

Nettle textiles were especially common in sixteenth- and seventeenth-century Scottish households, and were known as Scotch cloth. The English poet Thomas Campbell (1777–1844) wrote, "In Scotland, I have eaten nettles. I have slept in nettle sheets. I have dined off a nettle tablecloth. The stalks of the nettle are as good as flax for making cloth. I have heard my mother say she thought nettle more durable than any other species of linen."

The use of nettle fiber for clothing declined beginning in the sixteenth century as the cotton industry started to expand, cotton being easier and more convenient to harvest. In Poland nettle fibers were used until the seventeenth century, to be replaced by silk. By the late 1800s, flax and hemp superseded nettle because nettle needed to grow in rich soil and thus was more expensive to produce.

There was a brief resurgence of nettle fiber use during World War I due to a shortage of cotton. The Germans and Austrians collected almost 5 million pounds of garden and wild nettle to make uniforms when cotton, previously imported from Britain, was unavailable.

Nettle is being revisited today as a potential future fiber and dye plant because of its durability, environmental sustainability, and ease of cultivation. When nettle is spun into thread it is 50 times stronger than cotton and almost as strong as silk. When mercerized it is described as superior to cotton in making velvet. Nettle fabric, like cotton, can be dyed or bleached. The untreated plant fibers are a natural, camouflaging dark green color.

Making Nettle Rope

To make nettle rope, select the plants with the longest stems. Soak the stems in water for 24 hours, then lay them on a dry surface and pound with a smooth stone. Use a comb to separate the fleshy matter from the fiber. Dry in the sun on a hot day for a few hours. Twist or braid the fibers together to make a strong rope.

Nettle as a Dye Plant

Nettle is a natural dye plant that can produce beautiful colors ranging from a beige to light yellow with greenish undertones to a dusty green hue when iron (ferrous sulfate) is used as a mordant. Nettle roots mixed with alum produce a rich yellow dye that has been used to dye wool and Ukranian pysanky Easter eggs. Nettle was once used in the food industry to color canned green beans. The most vibrant colors result from using fresh shoots early in the season, and soaking longer deepens the color. As summer progresses, the colors will diminish.

Naturally Dyeing Wool Yarn with Nettle

Dissolve 1 cup alum and ¼ cup cream of tartar in 2 gallons water in a nonreactive pot reserved for dyeing. Dampen 100 grams of wool yarn and add it to the pot. Bring the liquid to a boil, then reduce the heat and simmer for 30 minutes. Hang the yarn to dry. The next day, mix 8 cups chopped nettle leaves, stalks, and roots in 2 gallons water. Boil for 1 hour and allow to cool to room temperature. Strain out the plant material, reserving the dye liquid. Dampen the yarn, add it to the dye liquid, and bring to a boil, then reduce the heat and simmer for 30 minutes. Rinse the yarn until the water runs clear and hang to dry.

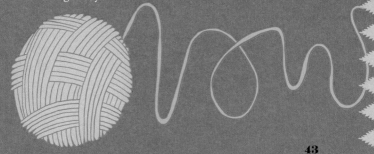

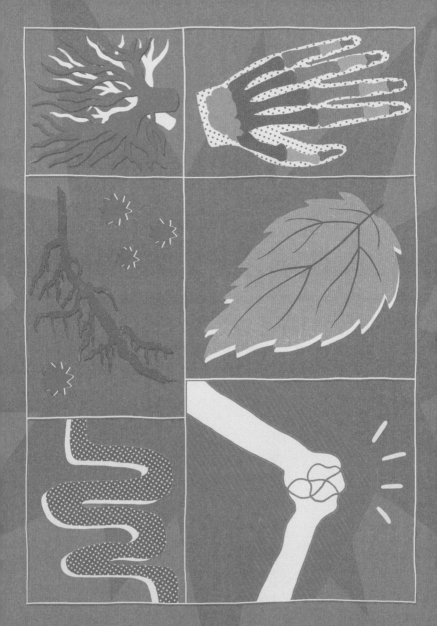

CHAPTER

NETTLE'S MEDICINAL PROPERTIES

As a therapeutic plant, nettles are one of the planet's most versatile and useful health agents. In herbalism, nettle is an alterative, meaning it helps alter or purify the blood by promoting the cleansing and healing action of the kidneys, liver, spleen, lymph, and bowels. It strengthens the adrenal glands and has a special affinity for the blood, bladder, and lungs. Nettle leaf and root tone or firm tissue, muscles, arteries, and skin. Nettles improve general weakness and anemia and are regarded as an anti-inflammatory plant due to the presence of caffeoylmalic acid and other phenolic acid derivatives that inhibit the biosynthesis of the inflammatory compounds leukotrienes and prostaglandins.

NETTLE REMEDIES

It would be challenging to think of another plant as healthful, useful, and versatile as nettle. From external to internal uses, nettle has helped humanity heal for thousands of years.

First Aid

Deters infection. Even before the discovery of bacteria, nettle was used to fight infection. Medical texts from the seventeenth century list nettle as an anti-infective agent. Nettle leaf and seed are indeed antiseptic, helping to deter the growth of bacteria, according to contemporary studies as well as folk medicine. Research finds nettle extract effective against the bacteria *Shigella* and *Staphylococcus aureus,* though *Escherichia coli* and *Pseudomonas* were not affected. A poultice of nettle mixed with salt has long been applied to wounds to deter infection.

Slows bleeding. Nettle is hemostatic and styptic, meaning it checks bleeding, tightens soft tissue, and improves blood clotting time. It slows and stops wound bleeding as well as excessive menstrual flow. During the Civil War, Confederate Army physician and surgeon Francis Peyre Porcher wrote a medical text titled *Resources of the Southern Fields and Forests*, in which he related how he and another physician cut open a major artery of a sheep and applied some nettle tea–soaked gauze to the incision to stop the bleeding.

Nineteenth-century French doctors reported that nettle was superior to ergot in stopping bleeding. Capillary bleeding due to excessive vomiting or heavy cough are treated by nettle steamed and served with apple cider vinegar. Nettle powder, made from the pulverized dried herb, or boiled leaves have been used topically to staunch bleeding wounds.

Uses of nettle's hemostatic properties have included snuffing the dried powdered leaves to stop nosebleed or applying a cotton swab soaked in nettle tea or nettle juice to the affected area to curb bleeding.

One teaspoon of the juice can be taken every hour to stop hemorrhage from the intestines, uterus, nose, lungs, and stomach. Nettle is a vulnerary, promoting wound healing. It even helps rebuild the blood after excess has been shed. Nettle is also a remedy for the treatment of swelling after an injury.

Helps repair bone fractures. When nettle is mixed with oatstraw (*Avena sativa*) and horsetail (*Equisetum arvense*) and taken several times daily as a tea or in capsules, it helps provide needed minerals for bone repair after a fracture. It can also speed the healing of tendons and improve connective tissue health. Cool nettle tea or lotion is used to soothe and heal burns, scalds, and sunburn.

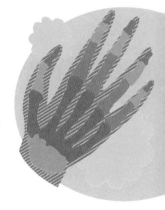

Blood Sugar Disorders

Animal studies indicate that nettle lowers blood sugar levels, which may make it beneficial for diabetics. Nettle is rich in trace minerals, including chromium, that help stabilize blood sugar levels. It is considered beneficial for adult-onset diabetes as well as hypoglycemia.

Respiratory Health

Nettle supports the lungs due to its high chlorophyll content, which helps the body better utilize oxygen. In the first century CE, Pedanius Dioscorides, surgeon for the Roman emperor Nero, wrote of nettle that they "fetcheth up ye stuff out of ye thorax." Sixteenth-century British herbalist John Gerard proclaimed, "The nettle is a good medicine for them that cannot breathe unless they hold their head upright." Nicolas Culpeper suggested eating the spring tops of nettle and "boiling the roots

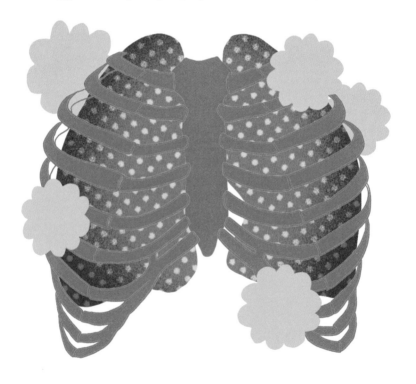

and leaves for easing lung troubles and pleurisy, also swollen throats and mouths."

Works as a decongestant. Its anticatarrhal properties help to break up mucus, and its expectorant properties facilitate the excretion of mucus from the lungs and throat. When used after a lung infection, the herb helps restore tone to the bronchial mucosa. Nettle is also considered a pectoral, or an herb to remedy chest diseases.

Contains anti-asthmatic properties. Nettle is used especially for asthma triggered by food or airborne allergies, less so for exercise-induced or inflammation-based asthma. At one time in history, inhaling the smoke of burning dried nettle leaves was a home remedy for asthma, congestion, and bronchial problems, due to the herb's antispasmodic and antihistamine effects. Nettle tea, extract, capsules, or juice are especially beneficial for heat-type asthma, which is characterized by red face, fever, rapid heavy breathing, yellowish mucus, scant urine, and dry stools.

Is antibacterial. Nettle seeds have traditionally been used in Europe and North America to treat consumption or tuberculosis, due to the herb's antibacterial activity against the tuberculosis mycobacterium. During medieval times the fresh juice was given to remedy tuberculosis. A form of scrofula known as cervical tuberculosis lymphadenitis (tuberculosis of the lymph glands in the neck) has also been successfully treated with nettle.

Allergies

Nettle is considered antiallergenic. A lab technician at the Eclectic Institute in Portland, Oregon, accidently discovered that taking capsules of freeze-dried nettles improved his hay fever almost immediately, which led to a 1990 study at the National College of Naturopathy. In an experimental double-blind study, 69 patients with allergic rhinitis were randomly given either a placebo or a freeze-dried preparation of *Urtica dioica*. Fifty-eight percent of the patients rated it as moderately effective, while only 37 percent of those using a placebo reported such benefit. Taking nettle before the hay fever season begins can minimize the annual discomfort of hay fever.

Nettle stabilizes the mast cell walls, which stops the aggravating cycle of mucus membrane hyperactivity and inflammation. It helps dry out the sinuses, especially when used in the freeze-dried form, and ameliorates allergic rhinitis by calming a runny nose, preventing excessive mucus production, and decreasing airway inflammation. In other words, it's a strong antihistamine. And its high content of beta-carotene and vitamin C strengthen mucous membranes.

Because it is a natural antihistamine, nettle is excellent when a patient has food or airborne allergies. Twentieth-century herbalist William LeSassier said that "Nettles are an excellent herb to make regular use of for people that have multiple allergies and also for people that are allergic to everything." Nettle improves the body's resistance to pollens, molds, and environmental pollutants. Nettle tincture, juice, freeze-dried capsules, or tea can be used. Nettle is even useful for itchy skin conditions and to ease food allergy reactions.

Bronchitis and Pneumonia

When nettles are used in a steam pot, they benefit both bronchitis and pneumonia.

Nettle seeds have been administered throughout history to help heal the lungs following bronchitis and to restore integrity to the bronchial mucosa. In Australia the juice of the roots and leaves is mixed with honey or sugar to relieve bronchitis.

Other respiratory ailments that benefit from nettle's decongestant and expectorant properties are catarrh, pleurisy, sinusitis, and poor oxygenation. Perhaps due to its silica content nettle is helpful for treating coughing blood (hemoptysis), whooping cough, and phlegm in the lungs.

Skin Health

Nettle leaf can address several skin problems as it aids in detoxification. It is used both internally and topically in salves and poultices for acne, adult and children's eczema, hives, boils, vitiligo, rashes, pityriasis (also known as "Christmas tree rash"), psoriasis, and athlete's foot. In Russia nettles are considered an official herb of dermatology.

Cardiovascular Health

Nettle can help lower high blood pressure and stimulate nitric oxide production, which has a vasodilating effect, helping the muscles of the blood vessels relax, widening them and thus improving circulation. Nettle is a blood builder that improves anemia. Its high vitamin C content improves iron assimilation. Nettle aids in the formation of hemoglobin in red blood cells. Tests in 1898 indicated that anemia cases that did not respond to iron therapy improved quickly when nettle was administered. According to Amanda McQuade, author of *The Herbal Menopause Book*, nettles help normalize blood quality.

A cardiac tonic. In Russia nettle is used to treat atherosclerosis, a form of arteriosclerosis accompanied by fatty degeneration, and to reduce cholesterol. Nettle helps restore the elasticity of the arterial walls, and as it shortens blood clotting time, it has been used for hemophilia.

Until the late 1800s, old medical texts described using nettle to treat conditions that today would receive heart transplants. The heart enlarges when blood is anemic, which nettle improves, thus nettle is one remedy used for heart enlargement. German studies in the 1980s found that nettle juice given to patients with heart disorders exhibited increased diuresis (production of urine). Buerger's disease (also known as thromboangiitis obliterans), which affects mostly men and is characterized by inflammation and narrowing of blood vessels of the limbs, causing blood clots and painful walking, has also been remedied by nettles. The *British Herbal Pharmacopoeia* recommends nettle along with yarrow (*Achillea millefolium*) and melilot (*Melilotus* spp.) to prevent coronary thrombosis.

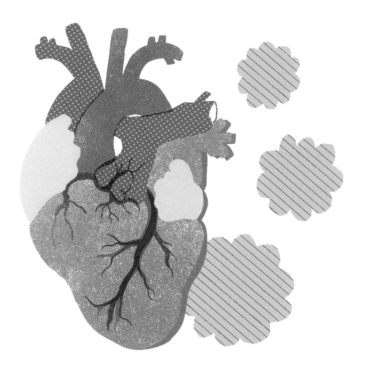

Nettle has even been used to treat congestive heart failure, by preventing fluid accumulation. Consult with a health professional, as this condition requires medical supervision.

Prevents blood clots and varicose veins. Nettle is considered a circulatory stimulant, helping to provide necessary minerals to the tissues. It can be used internally as food, tea, or capsules, as it nourishes and tones the veins, improves their elasticity, reduces inflammation, and helps prevent blood clots. Nettle and horsetail (*Equisetum arvense*) combined strengthen connective tissue, and can thus prevent and treat varicose veins. Applied topically as a tea, nettle aids varicose veins.

Digestion and Colon Health

Nettle leaf is considered a digestive aid and a carminative (something that relieves gas from the stomach and intestines). Nettle stimulates hydrochloric acid and bile production, which improves digestion and reduces digestive acidity and perhaps helps with the digestion and assimilation of protein.

Nettle works to clear mucus from the colon and gently stimulate the bowels. Nettle contains a substance called secretin; this causes the bowels to slough off their heavier mucus coating from a winter of eating heavy foods. Nettle also encourages the growth of intestinal villi. It may be of help to those with celiac disease because of this quality and the fact that it ameliorates allergies. Enteritis (inflammation of the small intestines) can be helped by nettle. In Europe and Asia, nettle is used to treat colon problems including colic, diarrhea, and constipation. The leaf and seed are considered laxative. A decoction of the leaves can be used to treat diarrhea and dysentery.

Nettle can help curb rectal bleeding, though if this persists for more than a week do get medical attention to determine the cause. As an astringent, nettle helps strengthen and tighten blood vessels and thus relieves hemorrhoids when taken internally and applied topically as a salve or juice. It is safe even to use for hemorrhoids that occur during pregnancy. Nettle also promotes healing and decreases bleeding of ulcers in the stomach and intestines.

Parasites

Nettle was recommended in England in the days of Culpeper as a remedy against worms in children. Herbalist LaDean Griffin includes in his book *No Side Effects* a formula to treat amoebic dysentery. Nettle has also long been a folk remedy for round- and threadworms. The seeds are considered a vermifuge and anthelmintic, meaning they help expel and destroy worms, and have been used to rid the body of parasites.

Fatigue

Nettle's high iron and other mineral content helps increase energy after chronic or acute illness. Because it stimulates lymphocyte production, it has been found helpful in treating chronic fatigue. Nettle has been used as a restorative, bringing vitality back to a part of the body that has become atrophied, inactive, or paralyzed, including after the use of anesthesia.

Thyroid Health

Nettle seeds are used as an endocrine tonic and remedy for goiter. Old herbals suggest using 13 nettle seeds three times daily. Nettle benefits hypothyroid conditions as the seeds are a metabolic stimulant, and it contains small amounts of iodine, which is important for thyroid health.

Liver and Gallbladder

Nettle is considered a cholagogue, meaning it stimulates production of bile, and is used to prevent gallstones. In Russia nettle leaf tincture is used to treat gallbladder disease and is being studied for its effects on hepatitis. On a deep level in the body, it helps the liver produce blood proteins.

Kidney Health

Nettle leaf and root have a stabilizing effect and improve the kidneys' ability to excrete metabolic wastes and remove uric acid. As nettle is a diuretic, due to its potassium content, it causes more frequent urination, thus preventing kidney stones. For the first few days nettle is consumed, the urine will be darker and have a stronger odor. In one study, patients using fresh nettle over a 14-day period experienced a significant increase in urinary volume. In another study, animals fed nettle excreted more urea and chlorides than those not fed nettle. All over the world, nettle tea is consumed to prevent kidney stones. Consider nettle for chronic bladder inflammation with mucus in the urine.

For best diuretic effect, consume nettle as a cold tea. Unlike pharmaceutical diuretics, which cause the body to lose valuable minerals, nettle provides the body with trace minerals and electrolytes and facilitates the transportation of nitrogen blood wastes. Dropsy, which is an older term for edema, is improved due to nettle's diuretic properties. In Germany nettle is used to treat urinary retention. Kidney diseases including cystitis, glomerulonephritis, nephritis, pyelitis, and pyelonephritis all benefit from nettle. Nettle leaf is considered lithotriptic, meaning it helps loosen, dissolve, and eliminate stones and gravel from the urinary tract; at the same time it strengthens the system.

Michael Moore, author of *Medicinal Plants of the Mountain West*, reports that nettle is an especially beneficial diuretic for those in a more "acid" state. It helps make the urine more alkaline, which is helpful as acidic urine can contribute to stone formation. People who are going off dialysis have found nettle seed an ally.

For Women's Health

Helps regulate hormones. In the absence of menses, known as amenorrhea, nettle can help regulate the menses by building the blood. As such, it is an excellent herb to give to young women during puberty as a daily nourishing tea.

Alleviates PMS symptoms. Nettle helps improve fatigue during the menses. Because it improves liver function, it can help the body break down elevated levels of estrogen that contribute to bloating and breast tenderness. James Duke, author of *The Green Pharmacy*, suggests mixing nettles with burdock root (*Arctium lappa*) for this purpose.

Reduces heavy periods. Nettle is astringent, and its vitamin K content can help curb excessive menstrual bleeding or bleeding from uterine hemorrhage, as well as build the blood to prevent anemia. Nettle improves blood clotting ability.

Improves overall health. Nettle is considered a beneficial herb for women going off birth control pills because it builds the blood and strengthens the kidneys. Nettle stabilizes blood sugar, nourishes the bones, reduces headache and fatigue, tonifies the kidneys and adrenals, and beautifies the hair and skin. It may even help prevent breast disease—including fibroids, as nettle improves lymphatic drainage. For this purpose, it is ideal mixed with cleavers (*Gallium aparine*).

Provides key nutrients during pregnancy. Nettle has long been considered a parturient, or birthing aid. During pregnancy nettle provides trace nutrients, including calcium and iron, that help prevent high blood pressure and edema—both factors that can contribute to a dangerous health condition known as eclampsia.

Strengthens the uterus. Because of nettle's hemostatic properties, it is also useful in preventing or stopping threatened miscarriage. In case of the membranes or water breaking too early, bed rest along with nettle tea (Susun Weed also suggests violet leaf) is helpful. Nettle also strengthens the uterus, and its high mineral content helps prevent muscle spasms and leg cramps. Nettle can help prevent excessive postpartum bleeding. In addition, drinking nettle tea daily during the last 6 weeks of pregnancy provides the baby with natural vitamin K should the parent choose not to give the baby a vitamin K injection right after the birth.

Improves the quality of breast milk. During nursing, nettle leaf is considered a galactagogue, meaning it can improve the quantity and quality of breast milk. It also provides needed nutrients for the mother so that she does not feel depleted in the weeks following birthing. Nursing mothers will also find that drinking nettle tea on a regular basis helps prevent cradle cap in their babies.

A must-have for menopause. During menopause nettle helps restore a woman who has lost excessive blood due to menstrual flooding and is a prime remedy for premature cessation of the menses. Its high mineral content strengthens bones and nourishes thinning, dry vaginal walls. Farida Sharan, author of *Creative Menopause,* calls nettle "the ideal menopause friend."

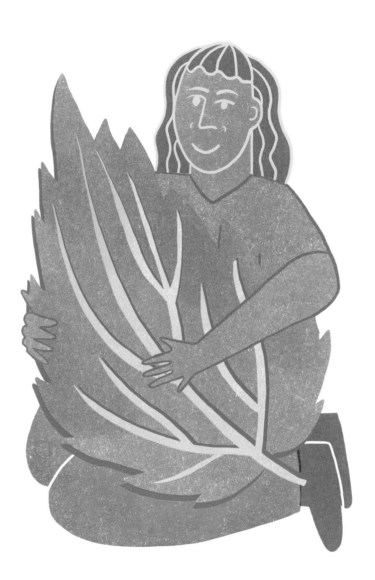

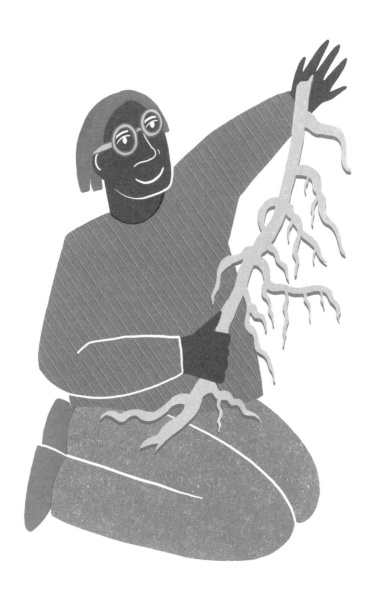

For Men's Health

Prostate enlargement, also known as benign prostatic hyperplasia (BPH) or hypertrophy, is often benefited by using nettle root as a tea, capsule, or tincture. Participants in a research project in France and Italy showed great improvement in BPH after using nettle for a month. At the Department of Phytotherapy in France, researchers found that nettle root was beneficial for mild prostate inflammation and a possible alternative to surgery. Nettle root inhibits the biosynthesis of DHT (dihydrotestosterone), which is a main factor in prostatic inflammation. Research in Germany, Japan, and the United States has established its value in treatment of benign prostate hypertrophy. Bazoton, a drug available in Germany for prostate disorders, is made from nettle roots.

In a French study, *U. dioica* and *U. urens* were administered to 67 men with varying degrees of prostate enlargement. Twelve of the men normally had to wake twice at night to urinate; of those, 10 no longer had nighttime urination. Of 27 men who usually woke to urinate three times, 13 no longer needed to do so, and 10 of them needed to void only twice. Four showed no improvement. The remaining 28 men, all of whom usually woke three times, exhibited little improvement. In yet another study, when men were given pygeum bark (*Prunus africana*) with nettle root, their prostate problems cleared up. Researchers are considering whether nettle is effective either by reducing the amounts of testosterone circulating in the blood or by inhibiting the enzyme that makes testosterone.

Nettle, especially the seed, has a tradition of being used as a remedy for erectile dysfunction, especially when due to low blood pressure. In the second century, the herbalist Galen wrote that nettle seeds "taken in a draught of mulled wine, they arouse desire." Two thousand years ago the Roman poet Ovid described nettle seed in *Ars Amatoria* ("The Art of Love") as a remedy to intensify sexual pleasure. Andrew Borde, physician to Henry VIII, wrote "yf any married man the whych would have this matter or desyre and can not throwe imbecyllyte use the act of matrimony . . . in the mornynge use to eat two or three new layd eggs rosted, and put into them the pouder of the sedes of nettles with sugar."

A study done at Budapest University tested males using a combination of nettle and oatstraw (*Avena sativa*) and found that the mixture increased their stamina, strength, sexual vitality, and testosterone levels. The same combination trialed at the Advanced Study of Human Sexuality in San Francisco on 40 men and women demonstrated it successful in stimulating sexual desire.

Genital Herpes and Warts
In the treatment of genital herpes and genital warts, diluted nettles tincture or fresh nettle juice helps dry the sores and relieves pain.

Fertility
Nettle can be a remedy for increasing fertility in both men and women. As a uterine tonic and nutritive, it strengthens the kidneys and adrenal glands. Herbalist Susun Weed, author of *Wise Woman Herbal for the Childbearing Year*, considers nettle her "second favorite brew for increasing fertility" right after red clover (*Trifolium pratense*). Added to fertility formulas with nettle have been milky oats (*Avena sativa*) and sea buckthorn (*Hippophae* spp.).

For Children

Nettle is considered a mild herb, suitable for use by children. It provides beneficial minerals to nourish their developing teeth, brain, muscles, and bones. It can be given for infant diarrhea. It is also an appropriate herb to use internally when suffering from measles or chicken pox, due to its blood-purifying properties. Nettle's rich supply of nutrients can even keep children's blood sugar on an even keel, preventing behavior problems and emotional instability.

Nettle tea given to children can be flavored with a bit of honey, some apple juice, a dash of tamari, or a natural bouillon cube. Health food stores also carry kid-friendly alcohol-free nettle tinctures formulated with a vegetable glycerin base. Nettle is also a traditional remedy for bedwetting, as it strengthens the kidneys and bladder.

Immune System

Nettle is considered an antioxidant and is certainly immune supportive. It aids the immune system with its tonic and alterative properties. Nettle has activity against candida. Use nettle when the immune system is stressed from dealing with Epstein-Barr virus, HIV, and chemical exposure. During the nineteenth century, nettle was recommended for people who were "constitutionally weak." A plant protein (lectin) in nettle leaf helps promote lymphocyte production. Nettle can be used to calm an enlarged spleen.

Nettle helps decrease susceptibility to colds and flus. It is a febrifuge, meaning it reduces fever, and can be given for sore throat and night sweats as well as for mononucleosis (a.k.a. glandular fever), which causes sore throat, fever, and fatigue as well as swollen glands. Nettle can promote recovery, detoxify the body, and improve energy. The seeds and flowers help ague, an old term for malarial fever. Drinking nettle tea before and after surgery builds the blood, promotes healthy blood clotting, speeds recovery, and helps you reclaim your energy. Nettle can be given to children and adults whose immune systems have been weakened by the overuse of antibiotics.

Cancer

Nettle is considered a depurative, an agent that cleanses or purifies the body. Any dark green leafy vegetable high in chlorophyll and beta-carotene is a good cancer-preventive food, and nettles certainly fill the high-nutritional profile. In recent years, nettle root has been used in Germany to treat prostate cancer. Twentieth-century herbalist Maria Treben (1907–1991), author of *Health through God's Pharmacy*, recommended nettle for leukemia and tumors in the spleen.

Nettle assists people receiving chemotherapy by protecting the blood from undergoing mutagenic changes. Since it stimulates hair growth, nettle can lessen hair loss caused by cancer therapies or enable it to grow back more quickly. Nettle's selenium content helps to prevent DNA damage from radiation therapy. During chemotherapy treatments, nettle can decrease fatigue, remedy fluid retention, prevent kidney and liver damage, and protect the veins. Nettle builds the blood and helps prevent bloating and erratic mood swings during the trying time of dealing with cancer. Indeed, nettle has been used as a traditional folk remedy for cancerous tumors.

Detoxification

Nettle stimulates bowel movements and is considered a spring-time blood purifier. Long regarded in Sweden as a spring tonic, nettle works to correct dietary deficiencies that develop in the winter months.

Nettle seeds are a useful antidote for spider, bee, dog, and snake bites, perhaps because the seeds are so detoxifying and improve the ability of the liver and kidneys to clean the blood.

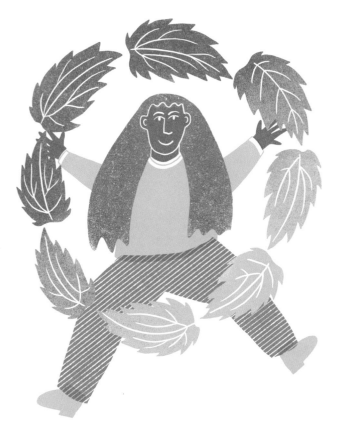

Pollution is another toxin that nettle deals with. For example, during the Industrial Revolution the English herbalist John Skelton recommended nettle along with other cleansing herbs such as burdock (*Arctium lappa*), cleavers (*Galium aparine*), red clover (*Trifolium pratense*) and yellow dock (*Rumex crispus*) to counteract "the constant deterioration of the blood from impure air and exhaustion by day, bad ventilation by night and want of attention to the ordinary requirements of life." It is interesting that all these plants that aid in pollution detoxification are themselves survivors—often growing in cities, near people— that have adapted to current conditions. It makes sense that as these plants have adapted, they can help us do the same. Nettle has even been used to help the body detoxify from arsenic contamination.

Pain Relief

In some cases, nettle can relieve backache, especially that associated with kidney problems. It has also eased sciatica. Taken internally as well as used as a topical compress, nettle can treat muscle strain and neuralgia. In Russia nettle is used as a remedy for pain, including toothache. The herb has helped headaches, including migraines.

Arthritis

Nettle is considered antirheumatic, benefiting arthritic and rheumatic problems. It decreases uric acid buildup when taken internally and increases circulation to the skin's surface. The most effective way to help arthritis is urtication with nettles (see page 76.) The Cahuilla people of California treated stiff muscles and rheumatism by stinging the soles of the feet with nettles. The Hesquiaht of British Columbia urticated with fresh nettles over arthritic joints and for stomach and back pain. In Germany nettle is included as a supportive therapy for rheumatic complaints. Nettles are also used topically as a poultice.

Emotional Health

Nettle is considered a nervine or restorative for the nervous system. Hildegard of Bingen, a twelfth-century mystic, abbess, and herbalist, wrote about nettle improving memory: "People who are forgetful against their wishes should take stinging nettles and pulverize them, add olive oil, and rub their chest and temples energetically when going to bed; this they should repeat, and their forgetfulness will decrease. The pungent warmth of the stinging nettles and the warmth of the olive oil stimulate the constricted vessels of the chest and temples, which sleep a little by waking consciousness."

Because nettle is rich in silica, which is a component of the nerve sheaths in the body, the herb can serve as a remedy for stress and nervousness. Combined with St. John's wort (*Hypericum perforatum*), nettle is good to add to herbal formulas for depression. Janice Schofield Eaton, author of *Discovering Wild Plants*, recommends nettle as a remedy for "the breakup blues." Nettle is also a traditional folk remedy for feelings of panic and powerlessness.

Nettle has long been suggested for people exhibiting poor concentration, poor memory, or dullness; difficulty getting up and being motivated; and excessive yawning or sighing. Nettle will put more pep in their step.

How Nettle Benefits Animals and Insects

Like people, animals and insects benefit from eating nettle. The stinging hairs of the plant also provide a safe place for a variety of living things to hide from predators.

As a Livestock Feed

In Victor Hugo's 1862 novel *Les Misérables*, Monsieur Madeleine (a.k.a. Jean Valjean) observes peasants collecting nettles and says, "When nettle is young, its leaf forms an excellent vegetable . . . chopped nettle is good for poultry, pounded it is good for cattle . . . the seeds, mingled with fodder impart a glossy coat to animals." An herbal research paper by Ferdinand von Mueller published in 1874 reported: "Fed a moderate quantity of Nettle seed for only 8 days, horses became fat and beautiful." During World War I, the German military instructions included feeding wilted or dried nettles to malnourished cavalry horses that had become thin and were suffering from digestive disorders.

Fresh or Dried

Only donkeys will eat fresh stinging nettles, but when the herb is dried, many animals will consume it with relish. Dried nettles are as rich in protein as dried cottonseed meal. Farmers wise to country ways, however, feed dried nettles as a dietary supplement to livestock, poultry, and pigs and add dried powdered nettles to pets' food. Chopped dried nettle gives a gloss to both feather and fur and a sparkle of health to the eyes, and it helps prevent disease.

In Sweden and Russia nettle has been cultivated as a fodder plant for cattle. Cows, sheep, and goats enjoy the taste of dried nettle, and it causes them to produce more milk. Chickens fed grain mixed with dried nettle are healthier, have increased egg production, and their chicks grow faster. Turkeys thrive and fatten on nettles. Chopped dried nettle can also be fodder for ducks and geese.

Pigs will eat boiled nettles. Nettle seeds when added to the feed of horses and dogs give them a glossy coat. It is also reported that dogs fed dried nettle are less likely to have rheumatism.

Food for Bugs and Butterflies

Nettles provide food for at least 30 insect species and are useful in the garden for attracting butterflies and moths. Caterpillars of red admiral and comma butterflies chew their way around the threatening nettle needles and depend on the fresh, succulent leaves that most larger animals shun. Peacock and small tortoiseshell butterflies—so lovely that they are referred to as "flying blossoms"—are entirely dependent on nettles. They lay their eggs on the leaves, and tiny black caterpillars emerge to feed on the plant.

As a Shelter for Small Creatures

Where nettles grow wild, they often provide shelter and protection for amphibians, ground-dwelling birds, and occasional rodents. A stand of nettles is also reputed to protect bees from being encroached upon by hungry frogs.

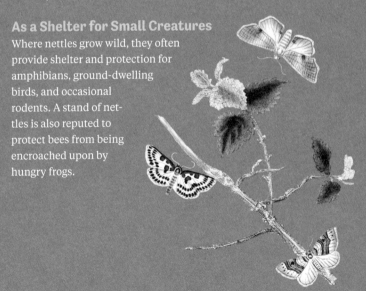

SOME THERAPEUTIC APPROACHES

Nettle also plays a starring role in a variety of other therapies.

Homeopathy

Homeopathy is a system of medicine in which minute amounts of substances are used to correct imbalances in the body. The homeopathic remedy *Urtica urens* is derived from the *Urtica urens* species of nettles and is available as a cream for irritated skin, burns, and bruises; tablets or pellets to take by mouth; and as a tincture taken internally or applied topically for bee stings and sunburn.

Urtica urens is used in the treatment of first- and second-degree burns and their resultant pain, as well as for chicken pox, eczema, edema, gout, hives, prickly heat, insect bites, and rashes, including those induced by shellfish allergy, those made worse by heat or exercise, and nettle rash. *Urtica urens* is also given for gout, rheumatism, neuralgia, and neuritis. For nursing mothers *Urtica urens* is indicated for low milk production with vulvar itching. It is also used for burning urine in cases of cystitis.

In general, *Urtica urens* is a remedy indicated when symptoms are improved from rubbing the area and lying down. Other factors in selecting *Urtica urens* are when symptoms become worse from exposure to cold, damp, or water and from being touched. *Urtica urens* as a homeopathic remedy is often recommended for symptoms that return at the same time each year.

Flower Essence Therapy

Flower essences are made by soaking the plant's flowers in springwater for several hours. The water is then collected and preserved, usually with a small amount of brandy. Flower essences are used to benefit the emotional body.

Nettle flower essence is recommended for angry, cold states that can lead to spitefulness and cruelty. It can encourage righteous anger and fearlessness in people who feel isolated or have been "stung" by others. It helps people regain the ability to connect with others by expressing necessary anger. It also helps release stress and is considered a blood cleanser and tonic. In doing this it helps reestablish harmony and unity. Nettle flower essence has been used for those undergoing the stress of a broken home and family, divorce, sibling rivalry, or adoption.

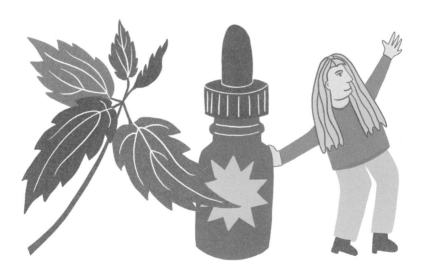

Traditional Chinese Medicine

Nettle affects the organs and meridians of the small intestines, bladder, and lungs. In Traditional Chinese Medicine, nettle is considered cool, dry, and astringent, with a slightly bitter and somewhat salty and bland flavor. It reduces heat symptoms. However, nettle also has many warming actions: It brightens the chi (vital force, life energy) and drains cold dampness due to its warming eliminative qualities. It nourishes the jing (essence, matter).

Ayurvedic Medicine

In Ayurveda, the traditional medicine of India based on mind-body-spirit connections that address specific body and energy types, nettle leaves and seeds are considered a rejuvenative (rasayana) tonic, especially for the adrenals and kidneys. Nettles are said to increase the vitality (ojas) and help those who are exhausted due to stress, illness, or old age. Nettle is considered astringent, cooling, and pungent. It nurtures the air element (vata) and decreases fire (pitta) and water (kapha) constitutions.

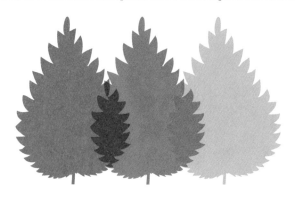

CONTRAINDICATIONS AND CAUTIONS

When used appropriately, nettle is considered safe, even over an extended period of time, although nettles should not be used for prolonged periods by those with overly cold, yin-deficient type conditions. Only the young tops should be used, as older plants can be irritating to the kidneys and may cause digestive disturbances. Do not eat nettles raw, unless it is done in the very earliest of springtime with the newest of growths, and then only with great caution. If you elect to eat raw nettles, make sure they are thoroughly blended or puréed. Note that eating raw nettles can cause digestive disturbances, mouth and lip irritation, and urinary problems.

Nettle tea is safe for long-term use. That said, excessive use of nettle leaf tea may cause skin rash, which should disappear when nettle consumption is ceased and plenty of plain water is consumed instead.

There have been rare reports of nettle root tincture causing gastrointestinal disturbances. If nettle causes a scratchy sensation upon urination, decrease dosages or combine with other herbs that are more demulcent, such as marshmallow root.

Stick with North American or European species unless you have consulted with local herb authorities on the safety of their local varieties. The *Urera baccifera* nettle that grows in the tropical Americas has a severe sting that causes considerable pain with numbness lasting several days. *Urtica ferox,* the nettle native to New Zealand, is so toxic that just five of its hairs can be fatal to a guinea pig. Massive nettle sting exposure has led to shock symptoms in some animals.

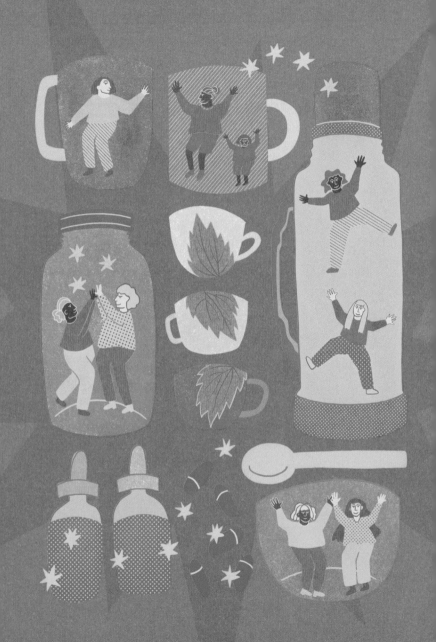

CHAPTER

4

MAKING AND USING NETTLE MEDICINE

You can prepare nettle by methods that are pleasant and effective. Nettle can be taken in many forms—as tea, tincture, juice, syrup, or capsules. Or maybe the best nettle medicine for you is through urtication—the deliberate exposure of skin to the herb's distinctive sting. There's surely a way to use nettle that suits your lifestyle!

BEFORE YOU MEDICATE, URTICATE!

Urtication is the practice of deliberately stinging one's bare skin with nettles, usually over an area that needs treatment, which causes a burning sensation. This practice has been followed for more than 2,000 years, since ancient Greek and Roman times, without any serious side effects. (Caesar's troops whipped their legs with nettles to numb them against the intense English cold.)

A Popular Remedy

Urtication has parallels with a form of bee sting therapy (apitherapy), in which someone deliberately receives a sting from a female bee, usually through a micromesh, so that the venom enters the body but the stinger does not imbed. Forms of apitherapy are currently used to treat pain and certain chronic inflammatory disorders. Like bee venom, nettles contain formic acid, which is considered beneficial in the treatment of many painful conditions. Today, nettle urtication is a popular remedy in Europe for the treatment of arthritis, burns, MS, musculoskeletal pain, Parkinson's, frozen shoulder, shingles, wounds, and other painful disorders. It's also a more environmentally friendly treatment than apitherapy, as it doesn't kill bees. Since many bees are dying due to mite infestation, insecticide, herbicide, and loss of wildflower habitats, bees need to be protected. (Yes, apitherapy results in a slow, long death process for the bees.) Additionally, some people are highly allergic to bee stings, which can cause anaphylactic shock. In contrast, nettles are cruelty-free, cost nothing if you gather them yourself, and are renewable and effective. Some people keep a few nettles in pots as houseplants so they enjoy pain relief even in winter.

How to Get Started

When trying urtication for the first few times, touch just a small area of skin and build up exposure gradually. Approach this treatment method with caution and respect.

To urticate, use fresh nettles. You can harvest them and place the stalks in a container of water until you are ready to use them. Begin by tying several fresh nettle plants together to form a bundle of nettles. If your legs, for example, are the problem area, brush the skin with the bundle, working first in a motion upward on the foot, up along the outside of the leg, and then down toward the foot. Repeat twice, then move the bundle from the hips across the bottom to the other leg, and repeat three times there. Use the nettle bundle in a similar way for other areas affected. Do not rinse with cold water for the rest of the day or the warm sensation will be replaced by a slightly burning one.

Alternatively, visit the plant directly where it is growing. It is easiest to cut a plant and give a firm slap to the area that needs a treatment, followed by a quick brush over the area. (You can go over acupuncture meridians, the soles of the feet, or any area that needs treatment.) This can be done for up to 5 to 10 minutes if desired, but most people will find just a few moments enough. Relief can last up to 12 hours.

How often should you do this? The recommendation is 3 days in a row, then a break of 3 days to prevent one from getting desensitized to the remedy. Continue the process as needed.

Health and Beauty

Over the past 50 years that I have worked with nettles, I have used nettle urtication in many ways. When I had a gum infection, I placed nettles between my cheek and gum and was able to avoid antibiotics. (I also used herbal antimicrobials such as myrrh.) I have had a lipoma on my neck for several years and after daily urticating, it has reduced in size by half so far; I will continue the experiment. When I had a bone spur in my foot, I placed nettles in my shoe and walked directly on the nettles, and the bone spur disappeared after a few days. And once I even had my massage therapist sting my entire body with nettles before the most excellent massage.

I'm not alone in experiencing benefits. My daughter, Rainbeau, an international activist, author, and model, has stung her thighs and buttocks as a way to prevent cellulite. A friend recently had hip replacement surgery and has been stinging the area where the incision was and has reported improved reduction of inflammation, less pain, increased feeling, and easier waking. And yes, I had a sweetheart (or two) brave enough to let me sting their privates with nettles (mine, too) and then having awesome, intense lovemaking right afterward, due to the increased circulation. A number of musicians and carpenters come over every few weeks to urticate their hands, fingers, and wrists to relieve the cramping from excess guitar playing or hammering. My German friend has told me that every spring her grandfather would disrobe, stand at the top of a nettle-covered hill, then roll down the hill as an arthritis remedy.

So, it bears repeating: Before you medicate, urticate!

TEA PREPARATIONS

Nettle tea was a popular beverage in eighteenth-century Paris, and it never should have gone out of style! "Wildman" Steve Brill, author of *Identifying and Harvesting Edible and Medicinal Plants*, describes the tea as tasting like "a strong stock of rich, deep, green plant essence." Nettle tastes lovely on its own but tastes even better with the addition of mint and a teaspoon of honey or a dash of tamari and miso. Nettle tea can be enjoyed hot or cold, depending on your preference and the weather.

How to Make Nettle Tea

It is best to not boil the herb when making nettle tea. Instead, bring 1 cup water to a boil and turn off the heat. Add to the water 1 heaping teaspoon of fresh herb or 2 heaping teaspoons dried, cover, and let steep for at least 10 minutes. (I like to steep mine overnight.) Strain before drinking. A cup a day all year round is an excellent tonic. Up to 3 cups a day can be safely consumed.

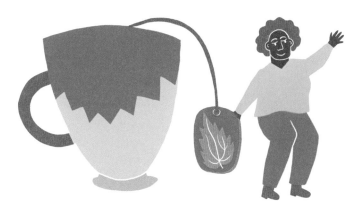

HERBAL TEA COMBINATIONS

Here are a few more simple nettle tea recipes with parts measured by weight. One part could equal 1 ounce, one-half part equals ½ ounce, and so forth.

To make the following teas, bring 1 cup pure spring, distilled, or filtered water to a boil in a pot. Remove the pot from the heat. Add 1 heaping teaspoon herb mixture to the water. Cover and let steep for 10 minutes. Strain and enjoy. Honey can be stirred in as an optional sweetener.

Bone-Strength Tea

1 part nettle (*Urtica dioica*) leaf
1 part oatstraw (*Avena sativa*)
1 part horsetail (*Equisetum arvense*)

Decongestion/Allergy Tea

1 part nettle (*Urtica dioica*) leaf
½ part mullein (*Verbascum thapsus*) leaf
1 part peppermint (*Mentha × piperita*) leaf
½ part fresh or dried ginger (*Zingiber officinale*) root

Energy Tea

1 part nettle (*Urtica dioica*) leaf
1 part yerba maté (*Ilex paraguariensis*) leaf
½ part peppermint (*Mentha × piperita*) leaf

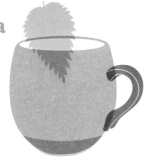

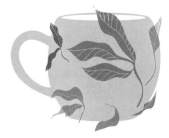

Healthy-Skin Tea

1 part nettle (*Urtica dioica*) leaf
1 part red clover (*Trifolium pratense*) blossoms
½ part dandelion (*Taraxacum officinale*) root
1 part burdock (*Arctium lappa*) root

Premenstrual-Blues Tea

1 part nettle (*Urtica dioica*) leaf
1 part red raspberry (*Rubus idaeus*) leaf
1 part German chamomile (*Matricaria recutita*) flower

Pregnancy Tea

1 part nettle (*Urtica dioica*) leaf
1 part red raspberry (*Rubus idaeus*) leaf
¼ part peppermint (*Mentha × piperita*) leaf

Nursing-Mom Tea

1 part nettle (*Urtica dioica*) leaf
1 part red clover (*Trifolium pratense*) blossoms
½ part fennel (*Foeniculum vulgare*) seed

OTHER WAYS TO PREPARE NETTLE

Nettles are used in everything from beverages and food to tinctures and syrups. Here are some easy ways to use nettles to heal common ailments.

Nettle Capsules

You can finely grind nettle leaves to go into pull-apart capsules. Powder the dried herb in a blender, a handful at a time, then fill both halves of the empty capsules and fit the halves together. Two size "00" capsules may be taken up to three times daily, as needed.

Nettle Tincture

To make a nettle tincture, place chopped fresh nettle root or dried nettle leaves in a glass jar and cover with vodka or brandy. Allow to sit for 1 month, shaking daily, then strain, discarding the plant material. Bottle the liquid in amber glass bottles and store away from light and heat for up to 5 years.

Be sure to label and date your tinctures—once arrayed side by side on a pantry shelf, they all begin to look alike.

For asthma and allergies, take 20 to 50 drops every hour until relief is obtained. For chronic symptoms, take 30 drops three times daily. As a hay fever preventive, take 30 drops twice a day for 3 to 4 weeks before the season commences.

Nettle Juice

Nettle juice, or succus, can be made by running the fresh, washed leaves and stems through a juicer. Before people had access to electric juicers, the leaves were wrapped in a wet cloth and gently heated for 30 minutes. Then the cloth would be wrung and the juice collected.

Use the juice at once or keep refrigerated and use the same day it's made. To preserve longer, mix 7 parts juice with 3 parts vodka (for example, 7 ounces nettle juice with 3 ounces vodka). If you want to avoid alcohol, replace it with vegetable glycerin at a rate of 6 parts glycerin to 4 parts fresh juice. Preserved nettle juice can be kept for about 6 months.

Mix the fresh or preserved juice with an equal amount of water and take 1 teaspoon at a time, three to four times daily. This dosage can gradually be increased to 1 tablespoon three times daily. It is an excellent tonic for anemia. It has traditionally been recommended for cardiac insufficiency with fluid retention. Some like to mix the juice with five times more buttermilk. Overdosing on the juice can cause diarrhea and vomiting, so use in small amounts as recommended.

One-half cup fresh nettle juice contains 167 mg calcium, 86 mg phosphorus, 3.2 mg iron, 72 mg sodium, 311 mg potassium, 4,715 IU provitamin A, 57 mg vitamin C, 91 mg bioflavonoids, 112 mg magnesium, and 7 mcg selenium.

Nettle Syrup

Nettle syrup is a delightful and tasty way to enjoy the rich nutrients of nettle. Collect young nettle tops, then rinse and chop. Place in a large pot with 5 cups water for every pound of nettles. Cover and simmer for an hour. Strain, then add 1 cup honey for every 2½ cups nettle juice. Simmer again for 30 minutes, cool, place in sterilized glass jars, and store in the refrigerator for up to 3 months. Drink one shot glass 1–2 times daily.

Nettle Herbal Elixir

There's no reason not to enjoy other healthful dried herbs along with nettle. Here is a delightful tonic.

3 parts dried nettle (*Urtica dioica*) leaf

2 parts rose (*Rosa* species) hips

1 part yellow dock (*Rumex crispus*) root

1 part dandelion (*Taraxacum officinale*) root

1 part dandelion (*Taraxacum officinale*) leaves

1 part burdock (*Arctium lappa*) root

1 part raisins

½ part dried organic apricots

¼ part cinnamon chips

¼ part dried ginger

Blackstrap molasses

Vodka

1. Place the nettles, rose hips, dock, dandelion root and leaves, burdock, raisins, apricots, cinnamon, and ginger in a large measuring cup and measure the volume. Transfer them to a large pot and cover with three times the amount of water. Bring to a boil, then reduce the heat and simmer for about 2 hours, or until the liquid is reduced by half.

2. Remove from the heat and let steep uncovered for 2 hours.

3. Using a fine-mesh strainer, strain the liquid into a large liquid measuring cup, pressing on the solids to extract as much of the liquid as possible.

4. Measure the liquid and pour it into a clean pot. For each cup of liquid, stir in 3 cups molasses and 1 cup vodka.

5. Pour into a bottle with a lid.

6. Store in the refrigerator for up to 6 months. Take 1 tablespoon daily as a mineral-rich tonic.

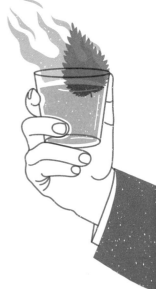

Plant Partners

Below are some of the herbs nettle is often combined with to address a particular condition.

Agrimony (*Agrimonia eupatoria*) herb as a spring tonic

Alfalfa (*Medicago sativa*) leaf as a mineral tonic

Cleavers (*Galium aparine*) herb as a lymphatic cleanser

Dandelion (*Taraxacum officinale*) leaf as a blood-building agent

Horsetail (*Equisetum arvense*) and **oatstraw** (*Avena sativa*) to speed repair of bones and connective tissue

Peppermint (*Mentha × piperita*) for a good-tasting mineral-rich brew

Plantain (*Plantago major*) as a pre- and post-surgery beverage

Red clover (*Trifolium pratense*) as a kidney or liver alterative, an agent that improves the organs' function

Tea (*Camellia sinensis*) as a stimulating beverage

Violet (*Viola odorata*) to treat skin rash

Yellow dock (*Rumex crispus*) root for acne, eczema, and psoriasis

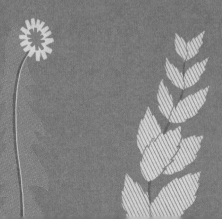

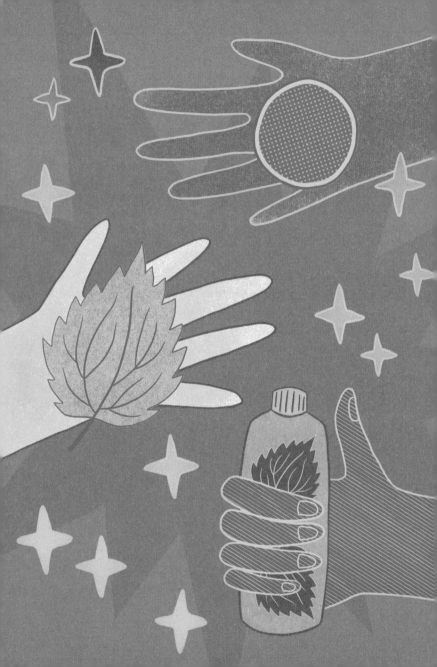

CHAPTER

COSMETICS

Long before commercial cosmetics were available, people relied on common herbs to enhance their looks. You may have noticed nettle as an ingredient in your shampoo, hair conditioner, or skincare products. Nettle's astringent and mineral-rich properties make it a tonic for the face, body, scalp, and hair. It helps balance oily conditions and deters fungal and bacterial growth.

NETTLES FOR BEAUTY

Drinking nettle tea nourishes the hair, skin, and nails thanks to the herb's excellent mineral and stimulating properties. When consumed regularly, it helps clear up dark circles under the eyes. The high chlorophyll content has natural deodorizing properties. Nettle helps curb the appetite, and cleanses toxins from the body. Since nettle is energizing, it helps in the motivation to stay on a healthy diet. It is used internally as a tea to remedy acne and eczema. Cold nettle tea is applied to relieve the pain and inflammation of sunburn.

For Hair

Nettle was frequently used by Roman and Greek beauties for long hair that shined. Nettle is acidic and helps normalize the sebaceous glands, making it an excellent conditioner or final hair rinse. It also helps to control dandruff—even stubborn cases—when used internally and topically. Root, leaf, and seeds are all used in antidandruff shampoo.

To treat hair loss, a tea, tincture, or juice of the nettle leaves and roots can be rubbed into the scalp daily. In France men often splash a combination of nettle tea diluted with apple cider vinegar on their scalps to prevent balding. Nettle leaf, seed, and root can also be taken internally to promote healthy hair growth and to deter hair loss and graying, due to nettle's rich pigment content.

Nettle-Rosemary-Sage Shampoo

This shampoo doesn't lather like store-bought ones with sulfates, but it does leave the hair feeling thick and looking shiny and can be used every day.

Makes 2 cups

2½ cups water

¾ cup soapwort (*Saponaria officinalis*)

½ cup chopped nettle leaves

¼ cup dried chopped rosemary (*Rosmarinus officinalis*) leaves

¼ cup dried chopped sage (*Salvia officinalis*) leaves

1. Combine the water and soapwort in a stainless steel pot. Bring to a boil, then reduce the heat and simmer for 10 minutes.

2. Stir in the nettle, rosemary, and sage. Remove from the heat and cover. Steep the herbs for 30 minutes.

3. Strain the ingredients through a fine-mesh strainer or several layers of cheesecloth. Compost or discard the solids and pour the liquid into a 32-ounce bottle. Store in the refrigerator for up to 4 days.

4. Shake well before using.

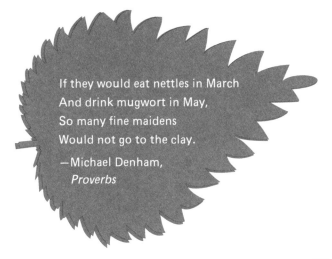

If they would eat nettles in March
And drink mugwort in May,
So many fine maidens
Would not go to the clay.

—Michael Denham,
  Proverbs

Nettle Hair Tonic

Makes 1 quart

1 quart apple cider vinegar

2 cups chopped fresh nettle leaves

½ cup dried rosemary (*Rosmarinus officinalis*) leaves

½ cup dried sage (*Salvia officinalis*) leaves

1. Combine the vinegar, nettle, rosemary, and sage in a jar. Cap tightly and store in a cool, dry place for 2 weeks, shaking the mixture daily.

2. Strain the mixture through a fine-mesh strainer or several layers of cheesecloth. Compost or discard the solids and pour the liquid into a 32-ounce bottle.

3. Massage the tonic onto the scalp before bedtime, then brush the hair well. Or use it as a final rinse without washing it out.

4. Store unused tonic in the refrigerator. It will keep for up to a week.

Aftershave

Nettle tea can be used as an aftershave lotion when mixed with equal parts witch hazel.

Calming Foot Soak

Austrian herbalist Maria Treben recommended nettle tea as a foot soak to prevent amputations, but it can also soothe poor circulation, corns, and sore feet, and remedy diabetic foot concerns. Nettle footbaths have also been used to treat rheumatism.

Evening Foot Soak

Makes 1 foot soak

1 cup fresh nettle leaves

2 cups boiling water

3 cups hot water

1. Steep the nettle leaves in the boiling water for 10 minutes.
2. Strain the mixture through a fine-mesh strainer or several layers of cheesecloth into a foot basin (discard the solids). Pour in the hot water.
3. Soak the feet for 10 minutes before bed.

Soothing Bath Tea

As a bath herb, nettle improves circulation and tones the skin and thus can address sciatica, poor circulation, and coronary artery constriction. Make a nettle tea by bringing 1 quart water to a boil, then stir in 4 large tablespoons of dried nettles. Remove from heat, cover, and allow to steep for 10 to 20 minutes. Strain the tea through a fine-mesh strainer or several layers of cheesecloth and discard the solids before adding the tea to the bath. (The plant material can cause irritation if it comes in contact with the skin.)

Alternatively, place two large handfuls of dried nettle into a crew-height or taller sock, then tie the ankle portion of the sock securely so no nettles leak out. Toss the nettle-filled sock in hot running bathwater until the tub is filled as desired. Turn off the water and allow the bath to cool to a comfortable temperature, then get in and soak.

Nourishing Face Mask

Nettles can be used as a nourishing facial skin mask. Mix 2 tablespoons powdered oatmeal with enough fresh nettle juice to make a paste. Apply to the face, leave on for 10 minutes, and then rinse.

Face Mask for Blemishes

This mask is designed to prevent blemishes and oily skin and to restore skin elasticity. Simmer 2 cups dried nettle leaves and 1 cup water in a covered pot for 10 minutes. Carefully transfer the hot liquid to a blender and purée. Allow to cool a bit. Apply to a freshly cleaned face for 10 minutes, then rinse and apply moisturizer if desired.

Oral Health

Nettle's high chlorophyll content makes its juice effective as a natural breath freshener. Nettle in mouthwash and toothpaste helps reduce plaque and gingivitis. Add nettle tea to an oral irrigator to strengthen and tonify bleeding gums. Gargle with slightly cooled nettle tea to soothe a sore throat.

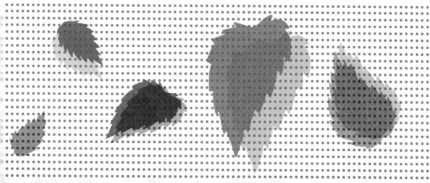

Compress

Compresses of nettle tea treat arthritic joints, burns, chilblains, eczema, gout, heat rash, insect bites, neuralgia, sciatica, tendonitis, and wounds. To make a compress, prepare a nettle tea, then strain the hot mixture through a fine-mesh strainer or several layers of cheesecloth into a bowl (discard the solids). Saturate a dry cloth, such as a washcloth, and apply the hot, wet cloth to the affected area.

Juices, Infusions, Tinctures, Salves, and Powders

In Jamaica, the fresh juice is applied to open wounds. Nettle juice can also be applied to warts and even poison ivy. To treat warts, rub the fresh juice on three or four times daily for 10 to 12 days.

The infusion can be applied to cotton swabs and used to stop a nosebleed. Nettle tea can also be used as a douche for vaginitis, an enema, or an eyewash.

Nettle added to salves promotes wound healing. Nettle salve can be applied to hemorrhoids.

Nettle tincture can be applied to contusions, sprains, swellings, and wounds.

Dried nettle powder can be mixed with honey and applied to burns, crushed fingers and toes, and wounds.

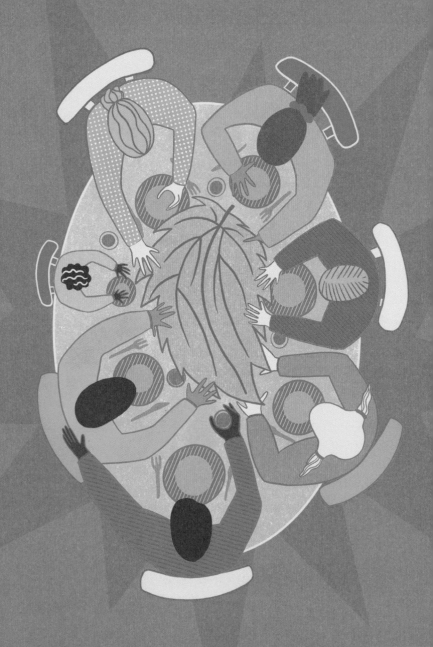

CHAPTER

COOKING WITH NETTLE

When it comes to cuisine, the nettle leaf reigns supreme. Nettle has a comforting, full-bodied mineral flavor and can be substituted in any recipe that calls for a leafy green such as beet greens, turnip greens, or chard. Nettle shoots can be boiled as a spring vegetable or steamed like spinach and served with a bit of olive oil. Nettle soup is most delicious. Nettle beer or wine is a favorite of many home brew aficionados and is often mixed with other wild plants like dandelion and burdock. In winter, when fresh nettle is not in season, many of these recipes can be made using twice as much dried nettle as fresh.

PREPARING NETTLE

Nettle must be cooked, dried, puréed, or juiced before it is safe to eat. All of the recipes starting on page 99 include instructions for how the plant should be prepared. To prevent unwanted stings, wear long rubber kitchen gloves when handling the fresh herb. Fresh nettle greens can be stored in a plastic bag or glassware in the refrigerator for up to a month, but once cooked they should be eaten within a few days.

Refer to Chapter 2 for detailed instructions about harvesting and preserving nettles.

NUTRITION

It is hard to surpass the nutritional value of nettle. "No other green vegetable excels the nettle in vitamin and mineral content," said herbalist Juliette de Baïracli Levy, author of *Nature's Children*. Nettle contains carotenoids (including beta-carotene and xanthophylls); vitamins B, C, E, and K; rutin; and bioflavonoids. Nettle is considered antiscorbutic, helping to prevent scurvy.

Minerals found in nettle include iron phosphate (helps reduce inflammation), magnesium phosphate, potassium phosphate (nourishes the brain and nerves), potassium chloride (breaks down fibrin), phosphorus, boron (increases estrogen levels in the body and helps the bones retain calcium), calcium, chromium, manganese, potassium, silica (strengthens the body's connective tissue), sulfur, and zinc (supports the immune system). Nettles are higher in protein than other green vegetables.

According to *Nutritional Herbology* by Mark Pedersen, the nutritional content in 100 grams of dried nettles includes the following. On the next page, you will see another table of nutritional values that comes from a different source. Just as two apples from the same market might vary in their nutrients depending on the soil and climates they were grown in, two nettle plants can vary in nutrients depending on when the plants were harvested and how much rain and sun were part of the growing cycle. Nature is always changing and never exact, and these two charts are provided to give a general idea of just how nutritious nettles truly are!

- ✿ Calories: 0.60 g
- ✿ Protein: 10.2 g
- ✿ Fat: 2.3 g
- ✿ Fiber, dietary: 43%
- ✿ Calcium: 2,900 mg
- ✿ Chromium: 0.39 mg
- ✿ Iron: 4.2 mg
- ✿ Magnesium: 860 mg
- ✿ Manganese: 0.78 mg
- ✿ Phosphorus: 447 mg
- ✿ Potassium: 1,750 mg
- ✿ Selenium: 0.22 mg
- ✿ Silica: 1.03 mg
- ✿ Sodium: 4.9 mg
- ✿ Zinc: 0.47 mg
- ✿ Manganese: 7.8 mg
- ✿ Beta-carotene: 15,700 IU
- ✿ Thiamin (B_1): 0.540 mg
- ✿ Riboflavin (B_2): 430 mg
- ✿ Niacin (B_3): 5.200 mg
- ✿ Ascorbic acid (vitamin C): 83 mg

Nutritional composition of *U. dioica*

Values are per 100 grams of dried nettles.

	DAILY VALUE (%)
Calories: 35	
Carbohydrates: 7 g	2
Fiber: 7 g	24
Protein: 2.4 g	5
VITAMINS	
Vitamin B_1 (thiamin): 0.54 mg	1
Vitamin B_3 (niacin): 0.4 mg	2
Choline, total: 17.4 mg	3
Vitamin B_6: 0.1 mg	8
Vitamin B_2 (riboflavin): 0.2 mg	12
Vitamin A: 2011.0 IU	67
Vitamin K: 498.6 μg	416
MINERALS	
Selenium: 0.3 μg	1
Zinc: 0.3 mg	2
Phosphorus: 71.0 mg	7
Copper: 0.1 mg	8
Potassium: 334.0 mg	9
Iron: 1.6 mg	9
Magnesium: 57.0 mg	14
Manganese: 0.8 mg	34
Calcium: 481.0 mg	3

(Source: NutrientOptimiser, 2022; NutritionValue.org, 2022)

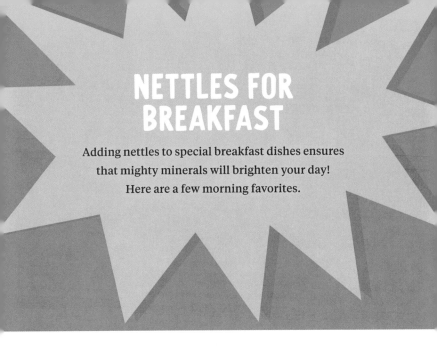

NETTLES FOR BREAKFAST

Adding nettles to special breakfast dishes ensures
that mighty minerals will brighten your day!
Here are a few morning favorites.

Fruit Whip with Nettle

Makes 2 servings

- 2 cups fresh nettles or 1 cup dried
- 1 apple, seeded and quartered
- 1 banana, cut into chunks
- 1 avocado, cut into chunks
- ½ lemon with peel, seeds removed
- ½ cup water
- Fresh berries, raw cacao nibs, or edible flowers, for garnish (optional)

Combine the nettles, apple, banana, avocado, lemon with peel, and water in
a high-powered blender and purée until completely smooth. Spoon the whip
into two serving bowls and garnish as desired.

Eggs Florentine in the Green

Makes 2 servings

- 4 cups chopped young nettle tops
- 3 tablespoons dairy or plant-based cream cheese
- ¼ teaspoon salt
- ¼ teaspoon freshly ground black pepper
- 4 eggs
- 2 slices whole-grain toast, for serving (optional)

  Salsa, for serving (optional)

1. Heat a lightly oiled skillet over medium heat, then stir in the nettles, cream cheese, salt, and pepper. Cook for about 3 minutes.

2. Make four little indentations in the greens and crack an egg into each spot. (The eggs will cook on the surface of the pan.) Cover the pan and cook until the eggs are done to your liking, 3 to 5 minutes.

3. Serve with a slice of toast and top with salsa, if desired.

Green Eggs, No Ham

Makes 2 servings

- 2 cups chopped young nettle tops
- 6 eggs
- 2 tablespoons vegetable oil
- 2 tablespoons milk or milk alternative
- ¼ teaspoon salt
- ¼ teaspoon freshly ground black pepper

  Whole grain toast, for serving

1. Whiz together the nettles, eggs, oil, milk, salt, and pepper in a blender until smooth.

2. Lightly spray a skillet with cooking spray. Pour in the nettle mixture and cook over medium heat, stirring every minute or so, until the eggs are scrambled. Serve warm with toast.

Nettle Popovers

Makes 12 popovers

2 cups young nettle tops
1 cup unbleached all-purpose flour
1 cup milk or milk alternative
4 eggs
4 tablespoons softened butter, plus more for serving
½ teaspoon salt
 Jam, for serving

1. Preheat the oven to 375°F (190°C). Grease the wells of a muffin pan and place the pan in the oven to get hot.

2. Whiz together the nettles, flour, milk, eggs, butter, and salt in a blender until smooth. Remove the hot muffin pan from the oven and fill the wells with the nettle mixture. Bake for 35 minutes, until puffed and golden on top. Serve warm with butter and jam.

Supercharged Recipes

Nettle is a true superfood, providing more benefits than most of the greens you can buy at the grocery store. Even better, nettles can be incorporated into a wide variety of delicious, healthy, and unique recipes! Whenever possible, I recommend preparing these recipes with organic, preservative-free, and cruelty-free ingredients.

Nettle Crêpes

Makes 4 servings

For the Crêpes

1 cup milk or milk alternative

2 eggs

¾ cup pancake mix (wheat-based or gluten-free)

1 tablespoon honey

½ teaspoon salt

For the Nettle Filling

1 tablespoon olive oil

6 cups chopped fresh nettle tops

3 cups sliced mushrooms

2 tablespoons fresh basil or 1 tablespoon dried

2 garlic cloves, minced

1 cup grated dairy or plant-based cheddar cheese

½ teaspoon salt

Chopped fresh parsley, for garnish (optional)

Make the crêpes

1. Whiz together the milk, eggs, pancake mix, honey, and salt in a blender.

2. Spray a skillet with cooking spray and heat over medium-high heat. When the pan is hot, pour in ¼ cup of the batter. Turn the pan to evenly distribute the batter. Cook for about 40 seconds. Flip the crêpe over and cook on the other side for another 40 seconds. Transfer the cooked crêpe to a clean dish and repeat the process with the remaining batter.

Make the filling

3. Preheat the oven to 350°F (180°C). Grease a 9-inch square baking dish.

4. Heat the oil in a skillet over medium heat. Add the nettles, mushrooms, basil, and garlic, and sauté for 5 minutes, stirring frequently. Stir in the cheese and salt and mix well.

5. Place ¼ cup of the filling mixture on each crêpe and roll each one. Place the crêpes seam-side down in the prepared baking dish. Bake for 15 minutes, until thoroughly heated and cheese is melted. Serve warm, garnished with parsley, if desired.

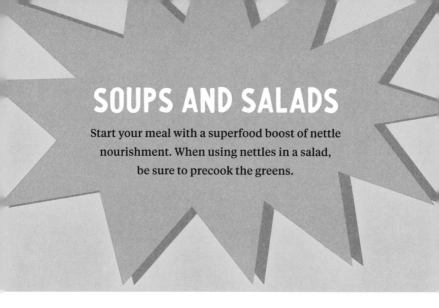

SOUPS AND SALADS

Start your meal with a superfood boost of nettle nourishment. When using nettles in a salad, be sure to precook the greens.

Soupe aux Orties (Nettle Soup)

Makes 4 servings

1 tablespoon olive oil

1 medium onion, finely chopped

1 garlic clove, chopped

2 teaspoons curry powder

2 cups chopped potatoes

4 cups chopped young nettle tops

4 cups water

Salt and freshly ground black pepper

Freshly grated nutmeg (optional)

1. Heat the oil in a soup pot over medium heat. Add the onion, garlic, and curry powder, and sauté, stirring constantly, for 3 to 4 minutes. Stir in the potatoes and nettles, and sauté for 5 minutes.

2. Add the water and cook until the potatoes are tender, about 25 minutes. Remove the soup from the heat and let cool for 10 minutes, then carefully transfer the hot soup to a blender and purée until smooth or somewhat chunky, as you prefer. (Alternatively, use an immersion blender in the soup pot.)

3. Return the soup to the pot to reheat. Season with salt and pepper and serve hot, garnished with nutmeg, if desired.

Chickpea and Nettle Soup

You'll need to start this soup a day in advance to allow time for soaking the chickpeas. Or, use two 14-ounce cans of chickpeas instead if you're in a hurry. Then skip to step 3.

Makes 6 servings

1½ cups dried chickpeas

12 cups water

2 tablespoons vegetable oil

1 tablespoon curry powder

4 cups chopped fresh nettle tops

1 (13.5-ounce) can unsweetened coconut milk

3 tablespoons lemon juice

2 teaspoons salt

Chopped fresh cilantro, for garnish (optional)

1. Place the chickpeas in a large bowl, cover with water, and soak overnight. The next day, drain the chickpeas and rinse well in a colander.

2. Transfer the chickpeas to a soup pot and add 8 cups of water. Bring to a boil, cover the pot, and reduce the heat. Simmer until the chickpeas are tender, 2 to 4 hours, adding more water if the beans look too dry. Drain.

3. Heat the oil in a large pot over medium heat. Stir in the curry powder and cook for 1–2 minutes. Add the nettles, coconut milk, lemon juice, salt, chickpeas, and 4 cups of water. Simmer, covered, for 30 minutes. Serve warm in bowls garnished with cilantro, if desired.

Salad with Nettles

Makes 2 servings

3 cups chopped young nettle tops

1 carrot, grated

1 hard-boiled egg, chopped

¼ cup olives or nuts (your choice)

Salad dressing (your choice)

1. Bring a kettle of water to a boil. Place the nettles in a large heatproof bowl, cover with boiling water, and let stand for 1 minute. Drain.

2. Stir in the carrot, egg, and olives. Serve warm, or let cool for 10 minutes if you prefer a cold salad. Serve with salad dressing.

Beans and Nettle Salad

Makes 4 servings

2 cups chopped young nettle tops

3 cups cooked kidney beans, black beans, navy beans, or chickpeas (your choice)

3 tablespoons olive oil

2–3 tablespoons lemon juice (from 1 lemon)

3 tablespoons chopped fresh parsley

1 tablespoon chopped fresh cilantro

1 hard-boiled egg, sliced

1 tomato, chopped

½ teaspoon salt

1. Steam the nettles for 3 minutes in a pan over medium-high heat. Transfer to a large bowl and allow to cool for 10 minutes.

2. Toss the nettles with the beans, oil, lemon juice, parsley, cilantro, egg, tomato, and salt. Refrigerate for 2 hours and serve cold.

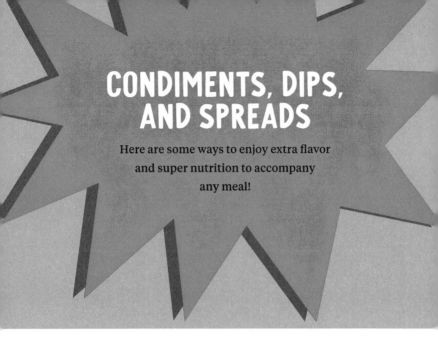

CONDIMENTS, DIPS, AND SPREADS

Here are some ways to enjoy extra flavor
and super nutrition to accompany
any meal!

Nettle-Sesame Sprinkle

I like to keep a jar of this in my fridge, but I also place some in a pepper grinder to have on the dining table. Use this sprinkle as a condiment on grains or vegetables.

Makes 1 cup

- 1 cup black sesame seeds
- 1 cup dried powdered nettles
- 1 teaspoon kelp

Heat a large skillet over medium heat. Toast the sesame seeds, stirring frequently, until they start to make popping noises. Remove the pan from the heat. Add the nettles and kelp and mix all the ingredients together. Let cool, then store in an airtight jar or spoon into a pepper grinder. It keeps for approximately 1 year.

Nettle Seed Gomashio

This is a delicious seasoning for soups and vegetables; I keep it on the table.

Makes 1 cup

1 cup sesame seeds
½ cup nettle seeds
¼ cup sea salt

Lightly toast the sesame and nettle seeds in a cast-iron skillet over medium heat, stirring frequently. Add the salt. Grind in a blender, mortar and pestle, or suribachi. Store in a glass jar at room temperature for up to 1 month.

Nettle Vinegar

Enjoy this condiment in salad dressings.

Makes 2 cups

1½ cups chopped nettles
1½ cups apple cider vinegar

1. Fill a pint canning jar two-thirds full with the nettles. Pour in the vinegar and stir carefully. Make sure the nettles are completely submerged. Screw on a plastic lid, or place a piece of wax paper under a metal lid so that the vinegar doesn't corrode it.

2. Set the jar in a warm place in the kitchen. Shake the jar daily for 3 weeks.

3. Strain out and discard the nettles, label the jar, and use within 1 year.

Sauce for Superheroes

Serve over baked potatoes, rice, or poultry.

Makes 1½ cups

¼ cup olive oil

1 onion, chopped

3 cups chopped fresh nettle tops

½ cup fresh cilantro or basil

½ cup water

½ teaspoon salt

¼ teaspoon cayenne pepper

1. Heat the oil in a pan over medium heat, add the onion, and sauté until transparent. Stir in the nettles, cilantro, water, salt, and cayenne. Bring to a boil, then reduce the heat and simmer for 10 minutes.

2. Carefully transfer the hot mixture to a blender and purée until smooth. (Alternatively, use an immersion blender in the pan.) Serve immediately. Leftovers can be stored in an airtight container in the refrigerator for 2 weeks.

Cheesy Nettle Spread

Makes 4 servings

3 cups chopped young nettle tops

1 onion, chopped

1 tablespoon olive oil

1 garlic clove

½ cup cottage cheese

¼ teaspoon salt

4 cherry tomatoes, sliced, for garnish

Whole-grain crackers, for serving

Whiz together the nettles, onion, oil, and garlic in a blender until smooth. Transfer the mixture to a serving bowl and stir in the cottage cheese and salt. Garnish with the cherry tomatoes and serve with crackers.

Dip-in with Nettles

Makes 2½ cups

2 cups chopped young nettle tops

1 cup plain dairy or plant-based yogurt

1 cup natural egg-based or plant-based mayonnaise

2 garlic cloves

2–3 tablespoons lemon juice (from 1 lemon)

½ teaspoon prepared horseradish

½ teaspoon salt

¼ cup chopped parsley, for garnish

Crackers, chips, or raw sliced vegetables, for serving

Purée the nettles, yogurt, mayonnaise, garlic, lemon juice, horseradish, and salt in a blender until smooth. Transfer the mixture to a serving bowl and garnish with the parsley. Serve with crackers, chips, or sliced raw vegetables.

Nettle Marinade

When nettles are marinated in vinegar, the formic acid is neutralized, making them safe to eat—and it's an excellent way to retain the nutritional value of nettle. Enjoy the marinade on salads or eat the nettles by themselves.

Makes 1 cup

Fresh young nettle tops

1 part apple cider vinegar

1 part olive oil

1. Pack a widemouthed jar with nettle tops.
2. Fill the jar to the top (no air space) with a 50:50 mixture of vinegar and oil. The nettles must be completely submerged.
3. Screw on a plastic lid, or place a piece of wax paper under a metal lid. Store in the refrigerator for up to 3 months.

SIDE DISHES

Why buy vegetables that are out of season
and trucked in from long distances when nettles
are ready to nourish you in every way?

Stir-Fry with Nettles

Makes 2 servings

- 3 tablespoons toasted sesame oil
- 2 garlic cloves, chopped
- ½ teaspoon grated fresh ginger
- 6 cups chopped young nettle tops
- ¼ cup water
- 2 tablespoons tamari
- Sesame seeds (optional)

1. Heat the oil in a skillet over medium heat. Stir in the garlic and ginger, and sauté for 3 to 5 minutes.
2. Add the nettles, water, and tamari. Cover the pan, reduce the heat to medium low, and steam for 5 minutes.
3. Garnish with sesame seeds, if desired.

East Indian Nettles

Feel free to add a protein of your choice to this recipe.

Makes 2 servings

1 teaspoon whole coriander seed

½ teaspoon whole cumin seed

1 teaspoon toasted sesame oil

4 cups chopped young nettle tops

½ cup water

Chopped fresh basil or cilantro, for garnish (optional)

1. Grind the coriander and cumin seeds in a mortar and pestle or blender.

2. Heat the oil in a skillet over medium-low heat. Add the crushed seeds and stir for 3 minutes. Add the nettles and water. Mix well. Cover the pan and let the mixture steam for 5 minutes.

3. Garnish individual servings with basil, if desired.

Creamed Nettles

Makes 2 servings

½ tablespoon ground coriander

1 teaspoon garam masala

¼ teaspoon freshly ground black pepper

¼ teaspoon turmeric powder

⅛ teaspoon cayenne pepper

4 tablespoons butter or coconut oil

6 cups chopped fresh nettle tops

3 tablespoons water

1 teaspoon salt

1 cup unsweetened coconut cream

⅛ teaspoon freshly grated nutmeg

1. Combine the coriander, garam masala, black pepper, turmeric, and cayenne in a small bowl.

2. Heat the butter in a pan over medium-low heat. Add the spice mixture and stir for 2 minutes. Stir in the nettles, water, and salt. Cover the pan, reduce the heat to medium, and simmer for 4 minutes, stirring occasionally.

3. Turn off the heat and add the cream. Garnish with a small dusting of nutmeg. Serve immediately.

Dumplings with Nettles

Use these dumplings in a soup or sauce of your choice.

Makes 12 dumplings

1 onion, chopped

1 tablespoon vegetable oil

2 cups rolled oats or leftover cooked rice

2 cups chopped fresh nettles

1 beaten egg, or 1 tablespoon chia seeds soaked in
2 tablespoons water for 10 minutes

¼ teaspoon grated nutmeg

1 teaspoon fresh sage leaves

1 cup unbleached all-purpose flour or gluten-free flour blend

1. Preheat the oven to 350°F (180°C). Grease a 9-inch square baking dish.

2. Sauté the onion in oil at medium heat for 3 to 4 minutes.

3. In a bowl, mix the oats, nettles, egg, nutmeg, sage, and flour, and then add the sautéed onion. Form 2-inch balls.

4. Transfer to the prepared baking dish and bake for 45 minutes, turning every 15 minutes.

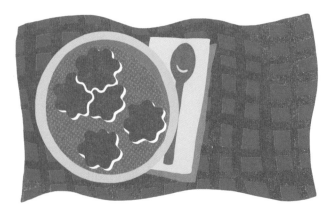

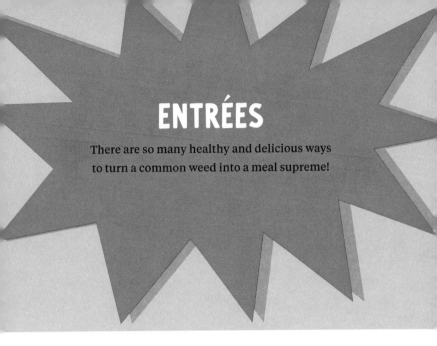

ENTRÉES

There are so many healthy and delicious ways
to turn a common weed into a meal supreme!

Pizza with Nettles

Makes 6 slices

- 1 tablespoon olive oil
- 2 garlic cloves, chopped
- 4 cups chopped young nettle tops
- 2 tablespoons chopped fresh basil
- ½ teaspoon salt

- 1 frozen pizza crust (wheat, gluten-free, or cauliflower-based)
- 1 cup grated parmesan or plant-based cheese
- 2 small tomatoes, sliced

1. Preheat the oven to 425°F (220°C).
2. Heat the oil in a large skillet over medium heat, then add the garlic and sauté for 2 minutes. Add the nettles, basil, and salt and stir for 5 minutes.
3. Follow the package directions for preparing the pizza crust, then cover the crust with the nettle mixture and sprinkle with the cheese. Top with the tomato slices. Bake for 15 minutes, cut into 6 slices, and serve.

Lasagna with Nettles

Serve generous squares of this lasagna with a side salad for a complete meal.

Makes 4 servings

1 tablespoon olive oil

6 cups chopped young nettle tops

3 garlic cloves, chopped

2 tablespoons fresh parsley or 1 tablespoon dried

2 tablespoons fresh basil or 1 tablespoon dried

2 tablespoons fresh oregano or 1 tablespoon dried

1 teaspoon fennel seeds

3 cups tomato sauce

6 ounces tomato paste

9 lasagna noodles

2½ cups ricotta or plant-based feta cheese

1. Preheat the oven to 375°F (190°C). Lightly grease a 9- by 13-inch baking dish with cooking spray.

2. Heat the oil in a skillet over medium heat. Add the nettles and garlic, and sauté for 3 to 4 minutes. Stir in the parsley, basil, oregano, and fennel seeds, and cook, stirring, until the garlic is cooked through, about 2 minutes. Add the tomato sauce and paste, and simmer for 30 minutes, stirring occasionally.

3. Bring a large pot of water to a boil. Cook the lasagna noodles for 5 to 7 minutes. Drain in a colander and rinse briefly with cold water.

4. Place a layer of noodles in the prepared baking dish, then cover with one-third of the tomato-nettle mixture. Dollop half of the cheese evenly on top of the sauce, then cover with a layer of noodles. Layer again with tomato-nettle sauce and cheese. The top layer is covered with just the tomato sauce. Bake for 30 minutes, until the cheese is melted and the noodles are lightly browned at the edges.

Spanakopita with Nettles

For a complete meal, serve a salad with olives alongside squares of this nutrient-rich riff on a tasty classic.

Makes 6 servings

- 1 large onion, chopped
- ¾ cup melted butter or olive oil, plus more for brushing pastry
- 8 cups chopped young nettle tops
- 2 tablespoons chopped fresh basil or 1 tablespoon dried
- 1 teaspoon dried oregano
- ½ teaspoon salt
- ¼ teaspoon freshly ground black pepper
- 1 box filo dough, thawed for 45 minutes
- 2 cups crumbled dairy or plant-based feta cheese

1. Preheat the oven to 350°F (180°C). Lightly grease a 9- by 13-inch baking dish.
2. Sauté the onion in the butter in a large skillet over medium heat until transparent, 3 to 4 minutes. Add the nettles, basil, oregano, salt, and pepper, and stir for 5 minutes.
3. Place 2 filo leaves in the prepared baking dish and brush them with melted butter. Spread one-third of the nettle mixture and one-third of the cheese, then add 2 more filo leaves and brush with butter. Repeat the layers two more times, so you have three layers of nettle mixture and cheese and four layers of filo dough total. (You may need only half the box of dough. Wrap the remainder well and refreeze or place in the fridge and use within 1 week.)
4. Bake for 45 minutes, until golden brown. Cut into squares and serve.

Pesto Presto Nettles

Serve on pasta, with crackers, or as a dip for raw vegetables like celery or cucumber slices.

Makes 4 servings

8 cups chopped young nettle tops

1 cup olive oil

½ cup pine nuts or walnuts

7 garlic cloves

½ cup grated parmesan cheese or nutritional yeast

Purée the nettles, oil, nuts, and garlic in a blender. Transfer to a bowl and stir in the cheese. Use immediately, or store in the refrigerator for up to 3 days.

Pasta with Nettles

Makes 4 servings

¾ pound capellini pasta (or gluten-free alternative)

2 tablespoons butter or olive oil

5 cups chopped fresh nettle tops

4 garlic cloves, chopped

1½ cups ricotta or plant-based cheese

3 tablespoons plain dairy or plant-based yogurt

1 tablespoon chopped fresh basil

1 teaspoon chopped fresh oregano

½ teaspoon salt

½ teaspoon freshly ground black pepper

1. Bring 3 quarts of water to a boil in a large pot. Cook the pasta over medium heat until tender, to about al dente. Drain and keep warm.

2. Meanwhile, heat the butter in a large skillet over low heat. Add the nettles and garlic. Cook, stirring occasionally, for 5 minutes. Stir in the cheese, yogurt, basil, oregano, salt, and pepper. Continue cooking for 1 minute.

3. Serve the nettle sauce over the hot pasta.

Pasta Casserole with Nettles

Give this casserole extra eye appeal, if you'd like, by decorating it with organic edible flowers like chopped marigolds or nasturtiums once it comes out of the oven.

Makes 4 servings

½ pound macaroni or small shell pasta (wheat or gluten-free)

2 tablespoons olive oil

1 onion, chopped

3 garlic cloves, chopped

8 cups chopped fresh nettles

¾ teaspoon salt

½ teaspoon freshly ground black pepper

1 cup dairy or plant-based feta cheese

½ cup pine nuts

1. Preheat the oven to 350°F (180°C). Grease a 2-quart baking dish.

2. Cook the pasta according to the package directions until tender, approximately 8 minutes. Drain.

3. Meanwhile, heat the oil in a large skillet over medium heat, then add the onion and garlic, and sauté for 3 to 4 minutes. Stir in the nettles, salt, and pepper, and cook for 5 minutes. Add the pasta, cheese, and nuts.

4. Transfer the mixture to the prepared baking dish. Bake for 20 minutes, until golden brown on top.

Calzones with Nettles

Serve with a side salad or some steamed broccoli.

Makes 4 servings

For the Dough

- 3 cups unbleached all-purpose flour
- 1 cup warm water
- 1 tablespoon honey
- 1½ teaspoons active dry yeast
- 1½ teaspoons salt

For the Filling

- 2 tablespoons olive oil
- 2 garlic cloves, chopped
- ½ cup chopped onion
- 5 cups chopped young nettle tops
- 2 cups ricotta or plant-based cheese
- ½ teaspoon salt
- ¼ teaspoon freshly ground black pepper
- ¼ teaspoon fennel seeds, crushed

Make the dough

1. Combine the flour, water, honey, yeast, and salt in a large bowl and stir until the dry ingredients are moistened. Cover and set in a warm place until the dough rises and doubles in size, approximately 1 hour.

2. Punch down the dough. Divide it into six portions and roll them into ¼-inch-thick circles.

Make the filling

3. Heat the oil in a skillet over medium heat. Add the garlic and onion, and sauté until translucent, about 5 minutes. Add the nettles and stir for 5 minutes. Remove the pan from the heat and stir in the cheese, salt, pepper, and fennel seeds.

Make the calzones

4. Preheat the oven to 450°F (230°C). Grease a baking sheet.

5. Place ¾ cup of the filling on each circle, being careful to leave a rim. Fold the dough over the filling to create a half-moon shape. Press down on the edges of the rim with a fork to seal.

6. Transfer the calzones to the prepared baking sheet and bake for 10 minutes, then flip the calzones and bake for 10 minutes longer.

Irish Stew

Makes 6 servings

- 1 tablespoon olive oil
- 2 medium onions, chopped
- 2 tablespoons chopped fresh thyme
- 1 tablespoon chopped fresh rosemary
- 1 pound cubed lamb or tempeh
- 3 carrots, sliced
- 2 medium potatoes, cubed
- 2 cups chopped young nettle tops
- 3 tablespoons unbleached all-purpose flour or gluten-free flour blend
- 2 tablespoons nutritional yeast
- 2 cups water
- 1 (8-ounce) bag frozen peas
- 1 teaspoon salt
- 1 teaspoon freshly ground black pepper
- 1 tablespoon chopped fresh parsley, for garnish (optional)

1. Heat the oil in a large soup pot over medium heat. Add the onions and sauté until translucent. Add the thyme and rosemary, and stir for 3 to 5 minutes. Add the lamb or tempeh, carrots, potatoes, and nettles, and cook, stirring often, until the lamb or tempeh is browned, about 5 minutes.

2. Mix in the flour and nutritional yeast, then gradually add the water, stirring continuously until the liquid thickens slightly. Bring to a boil, reduce the heat, and simmer for 1 hour.

3. Add the peas, salt, and pepper. Cook for 2–3 minutes. Serve in bowls and garnish with some of the parsley, if desired.

Potato-Nettle Curry

Makes 2 servings

1½ teaspoons vegetable oil

2 garlic cloves, chopped

1 teaspoon curry powder

4 cups chopped young nettle tops

3 medium potatoes, cut into ½-inch cubes

2 cups water

1 teaspoon salt

Chopped fresh basil or cilantro, for garnish (optional)

1. Heat the oil in a large saucepan over medium-low heat. Add the garlic and curry powder, and sauté, stirring, for 2 to 3 minutes.

2. Stir in the nettles, potatoes, water, and salt. Cover and cook for 20 minutes. Serve hot in bowls, garnished with basil, if desired.

Tofu with Nettles

Makes 2 servings

1 tablespoon toasted sesame oil

3 garlic cloves, chopped

½ pound firm tofu, cut into ½-inch cubes

3 cups chopped young nettle tops

1 tablespoon tamari

1 tablespoon chopped fresh cilantro, basil, or parsley (optional)

Heat the oil in a skillet over medium heat. Add the garlic and cook for 2 minutes. Reduce the heat to medium low. Add the tofu, nettles, and tamari, cover, and simmer for 15 minutes. Garnish each serving with ½ tablespoon of the cilantro, if desired.

Loaf Around with Nettle

Makes 4 servings

- 2 tablespoons butter or olive oil
- 1 onion, chopped
- 2 garlic cloves, chopped
- 6 cups chopped young nettle tops
- ¼ cup water
- 2 cups cooked white or brown rice
- 3 eggs, or 3 teaspoons chia seeds soaked in 9 tablespoons water for 10 minutes
- 1 medium tomato, sliced, for garnish

1. Preheat the oven to 375°F (190°C). Grease a bread loaf pan.

2. Heat the butter in a large skillet over medium heat. Add the onion and garlic, and sauté for 3 to 5 minutes. Stir in the nettles and water, and cook for 3 minutes. Mix in the rice and eggs.

3. Transfer the mixture to the prepared pan and bake for 30 minutes. Let cool for 10 minutes. Garnish with the tomato slices before serving.

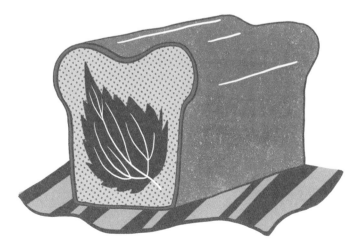

Ring Around the Nettles

Makes 4 servings

3 cups chopped fresh nettle tops

3 tablespoons butter or olive oil

1 onion, chopped

3 tablespoons unbleached all-purpose flour or gluten-free flour blend

1 cup milk or milk alternative

3 eggs, beaten, or 3 tablespoons chia seeds soaked in 9 tablespoons water for 10 minutes

½ teaspoon sage

½ teaspoon salt

¼ teaspoon freshly ground black pepper

½ cup grated dairy or plant-based cheese

1. Preheat the oven to 350°F (180°C). Grease a 10-inch ring pan.

2. Purée the nettles in a blender.

3. Heat the butter in a saucepan over medium heat, then add the onion and sauté for 3 minutes. Stir in the flour and gradually add the milk. Heat, stirring, for 2 minutes, then add the nettles.

4. Remove the pan from the heat and stir in the eggs. Add the sage, salt, and pepper. Cool for 5 minutes, then mix in the cheese.

5. Transfer the mixture to the prepared pan and bake for 35 minutes. Let the loaf cool slightly before loosening the edges with a knife. Remove from the pan by carefully flipping the loaf onto a serving platter.

Patties with a Purpose

Makes 4 patties

- 3 cups cubed potatoes
- 2 cups chopped young nettle tops
- 1 onion, chopped
- ½ cup raw sunflower seeds
- 3 tablespoons nutritional yeast
- 2 tablespoons coconut oil
- 1 egg, or 1 tablespoon chia seeds soaked in 3 tablespoons water for 10 minutes
- 1 teaspoon salt
- ½ teaspoon fresh or dried rosemary
- 1 red bell pepper, chopped, for garnish

1. Place the potatoes in a large saucepan and cover with water. Bring to a boil, reduce the heat to a simmer, and cook the potatoes until tender, about 15 minutes. Drain, return the potatoes to the pan, and mash.

2. Meanwhile, preheat the oven to 400°F (200°C). Grease a baking sheet.

3. Stir the nettles, onion, sunflower seeds, nutritional yeast, oil, egg, salt, and rosemary into the potatoes. Shape the mixture into patties approximately 4 inches around and place on the prepared baking sheet.

4. Bake for 30 minutes or until browned, flipping the patties after 15 minutes. Garnish each patty with 1 tablespoon of the bell pepper.

Soufflé aux Orties

Orties is French for "nettles."

Makes 6 mini soufflés

- 4 cups chopped young nettle tops
- 1 cup milk or milk alternative
- ¼ cup grated dairy or plant-based cheese
- 4 eggs, separated
- 3 tablespoons olive oil
- 3 tablespoons unbleached all-purpose flour
- 3 tablespoons nutritional yeast
- ½ teaspoon grated nutmeg
- ¼ teaspoon salt
- 6 cherry tomatoes, sliced, for garnish (optional)

1. Preheat the oven to 375°F (190°C). Grease six (6-ounce) custard cups and set on a baking tray.

2. Combine the nettles, milk, cheese, egg yolks, oil, flour, nutritional yeast, nutmeg, and salt in a blender. Purée until smooth.

3. Using a hand or stand mixer, beat the egg whites to stiff peaks. Fold into the nettle mixture.

4. Scrape the mixture into the prepared custard cups and slide the tray into the oven. Bake for 40 minutes, until golden on top. Serve warm garnished with sliced cherry tomatoes, if desired.

Potato-Nettle Bake

Makes 4 servings

5 potatoes, thinly sliced

4 cups chopped young nettle tops

1 onion, sliced

3 tablespoons butter or olive oil

1 teaspoon grated nutmeg

1 teaspoon fresh rosemary or
½ teaspoon dried

Salt and freshly ground black
pepper

2 cups milk or milk alternative

1. Preheat the oven to 350°F (180° C). Grease an 8-inch casserole dish with cooking spray.

2. Layer the potato slices, nettles, onion slices, and butter in the prepared casserole dish.

3. Sprinkle on the nutmeg and rosemary, season with salt and pepper, and pour the milk into the dish.

4. Bake for 1 hour, or until golden. Let cool before serving.

Rice with Nettles

Makes 6 servings

3 tablespoons vegetable oil

1 large onion, chopped

4 cups chopped young nettle tops

4 cups cooked basmati or brown rice

1 teaspoon salt

3 tablespoons chopped fresh parsley, for garnish (optional)

1. Heat the oil in a skillet over medium heat. Add the onion and sauté until transparent, about 4 minutes. Add the nettles and cook for 4 minutes. Stir.

2. Mix in the rice and salt. Stir for 3 minutes until warmed through.

3. Garnish each serving with ½ tablespoon of parsley, if desired.

Rice Balls with Nettles

Serve with a side dish of your green vegetable of choice, such as asparagus, zucchini, or broccoli.

Makes 6 servings

- 1 tablespoon olive oil
- 1 onion, finely chopped
- 6 cups chopped young nettle tops
- 2 cups cooked basmati rice
- 3 tablespoons almond butter
- 2 teaspoons dried sage
- 1 teaspoon salt
- ¼ teaspoon freshly ground black pepper
- 1 cup breadcrumbs (wheat-based or gluten-free)

1. Preheat the oven to 375°F (190°C). Grease a baking sheet.
2. Heat the oil in a large skillet over medium heat. Add the onion and sauté for 3 minutes. Stir in the nettles and cook for 5 minutes.
3. Transfer the nettle mixture to a large mixing bowl. Add the rice, almond butter, sage, salt, and pepper, stirring well.
4. Pour the breadcrumbs into a shallow bowl. With damp hands, form the nettle mixture into balls, using about ¼ cup of the mixture for each ball. Roll in the breadcrumbs and place on the prepared baking sheet.
5. Bake for 30 minutes, stirring the balls every 10 minutes so they brown evenly.

Loaf au Nettles

Makes 4 servings

- 3 tablespoons olive oil or butter
- 1 large onion, chopped
- 2 garlic cloves, chopped
- 4 cups chopped young nettle tops
- 1½ cups grated dairy or plant-based cheese
- 1 cup milk or milk alternative
- ¼ cup fresh parsley, chopped
- 4 eggs, or 4 tablespoons chia seeds soaked in ¾ cup water for 10 minutes
- ¼ cup raw sunflower seeds
- 1 teaspoon salt
- ¼ teaspoon grated nutmeg

1. Preheat the oven to 350°F (180°C). Grease a loaf pan.
2. Heat the oil in a large skillet over medium heat. Add the onion and garlic, and sauté until transparent. Stir in the nettles and cook for 3 minutes.
3. Remove the pan from the heat. Mix in the cheese, milk, parsley, eggs, sunflower seeds, salt, and nutmeg. Transfer the mixture to the prepared pan and bake for 35 minutes. Cut into slices and serve warm.

Spring Quiche

Makes 6 servings

For the Crust

½ cup vegetable oil

 2 tablespoons milk or milk alternative

¾ cup unbleached all-purpose flour or gluten-free flour blend

¾ cup cornmeal

 1 tablespoon dried sage

½ teaspoon salt

¼ teaspoon freshly ground black pepper

For the Filling

 1 tablespoon vegetable oil

 1 medium onion, chopped

 1 cup grated dairy or plant-based cheese

2½ cups chopped young nettle tops

 2 eggs or one (14-ounce) block of firm tofu

½ teaspoon salt

½ teaspoon freshly ground black pepper

Make the crust

1. Preheat the oven to 425°F (220°C).

2. Mix together the oil and milk in a large bowl, then add the flour, cornmeal, sage, salt, and pepper and stir until the dry ingredients are moistened.

3. Press the dough into a 10-inch pie pan. Bake for 5 minutes; set aside. Reduce the oven temperature to 325°F (160°C).

Make the filling

4. Heat the oil in a skillet over medium heat. Add the onion and lightly sauté for three minutes or until softened. Transfer the onion to the prebaked pie shell. Add the cheese and nettles.

5. Mix the eggs, salt, and pepper in a blender, then pour into the shell. Bake for 35 minutes, until the filling appears firm. Let stand for a few minutes before slicing and serving.

Noodles with Nettle

For this recipe, you'll need a pasta maker.

Makes 8 servings

 2 cups dried nettles

 5 eggs

 1 tablespoon vegetable oil

 ½ teaspoon salt

4½ cups unbleached all-purpose flour, plus more as needed

1. Powder the dried nettles in a blender. In a bowl, add 2–3 tablespoons of water to moisten.

2. Place the moistened nettles, eggs, oil, and salt in a blender and blend until smooth.

3. Transfer mixture to a bowl. Add enough flour to make a stiff dough. Knead on a floured surface until it doesn't tear when stretched. Cover and place in the refrigerator for 30 minutes.

4. Extrude the dough through a pasta maker according to the manufacturer's directions, adding more flour if needed.

5. Cook the fresh pasta immediately in boiling water until al dente. Alternatively, to enjoy the pasta later, dry on a baking sheet, on top of a clean cloth towel, or hang from a drying rack for 12 to 24 hours.

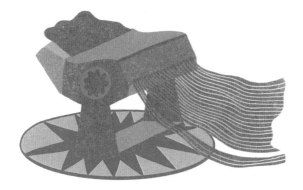

Pudding with Nettles

This is not a dessert, it's a main dish. It's extra tasty served with butter or gravy. Note that you'll need a paint strainer bag and a steamer for this recipe.

Makes 12 servings

16 cups chopped young nettle tops
 1 head broccoli, chopped
 1 small head cabbage, chopped
 2 medium onions, chopped
 ½ cup rolled oats

1. Mix together the nettles, broccoli, cabbage, onions, and oats in a bowl, then transfer to a large greased loaf pan.
2. Place the pan in a gallon-size paint strainer bag and tie it tightly with string. Set the pan in a steamer and steam for 30 minutes. Cool slightly to avoid burning yourself and place the pudding onto a serving dish. Serve in slices.

NETTLE BAKED GOODS

Powder dried nettles in a blender to add beautiful color and fiber.

Cheese-Nettle Biscuits

Makes 12 biscuits

- 2 cups unbleached all-purpose flour or gluten-free flour blend
- 1 tablespoon baking powder
- 1 teaspoon salt
- ¾ cups grated dairy or plant-based cheese
- ¼ cup finely chopped young nettle tops
- ¼ cup vegetable oil
- 1 cup dairy or plant-based milk
- 2 tablespoons melted butter or olive oil

1. Preheat the oven to 450°F (230°C).

2. Combine the flour, baking powder, and salt in a large bowl. Add the cheese, nettles, and vegetable oil, stirring with a fork. Add the milk and stir until the dry ingredients are moistened.

3. Dump the dough onto a lightly floured surface and roll it out with a rolling pin until it's ½ inch thick. Using a 2-inch jar lid or cookie cutter, cut 12 rounds. Place them on an ungreased cookie sheet and brush the tops with the melted butter.

4. Bake for 12 to 15 minutes, until golden brown. Serve warm.

Nettle Bread

Slice and serve with butter and jam, use for sandwiches, or toast it for breakfast!

Makes 1 loaf

- ½ cup warm water
- 2 tablespoons active dry yeast
- 1 tablespoon honey
- 1½ cups hot water
- 1 cup yellow cornmeal
- 2 tablespoons vegetable oil
- 1½ teaspoons salt
- 2 cups whole-wheat flour
- 2 cups unbleached all-purpose flour
- 4 cups dried nettles, powdered in a blender

1. Combine the warm water, yeast, and honey in a medium bowl and let stand until the mixture foams up, approximately 1 hour.

2. In a large bowl, combine the hot water, cornmeal, oil, and salt. When the mixture has cooled to lukewarm, stir in the yeast mixture. Add the flours, 1 cup at a time, kneading the mixture to combine the ingredients. Knead in the powdered nettles.

3. Turn out the dough onto a cutting board or clean countertop and knead for 3 minutes. Transfer to a large oiled bowl and cover with a clean towel. Allow to rise in a warm place until it has tripled in size, about 40 minutes.

4. Preheat the oven to 450°F (230°C). Grease a loaf pan.

5. Beat down the dough, shape into a loaf, and place in the prepared loaf pan. Cover, set in a warm place, and let rise for 15 minutes.

6. Bake for 10 minutes, then reduce the heat to 350°F (180°C) and bake for 50 minutes longer. Let the pan rest on a wire rack for 10 minutes before removing the loaf. For best slicing, let the bread cool before cutting.

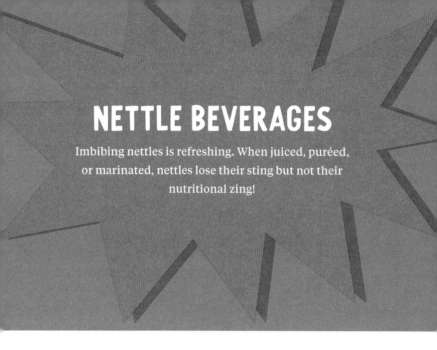

NETTLE BEVERAGES

Imbibing nettles is refreshing. When juiced, puréed, or marinated, nettles lose their sting but not their nutritional zing!

Wild Weed Juice

Here's a juice you can prepare without a juicer. I use a paint-strainer bag, available at any hardware store; just be sure to wash the bag first. Several layers of cheesecloth will also work.

Makes about 1 quart

- 2 cups fresh nettle tops
- 1 apple, quartered
- ½ unpeeled lemon
- 4 cups spring or filtered water

1. Combine the nettles, apple, lemon, and water in a blender.
2. Strain the mixture through a paint-strainer bag, squeezing to release all the goodness. Enjoy the juice immediately or refrigerate in a jar and enjoy the next day. Shake before serving. Add the pulp to your compost as an accelerator.

Nettle Vegetable Juice

For this nutrient-dense recipe, first run fresh beets, carrots, and nettles through a juicer and then measure the needed amounts.

Makes 2 servings

½ cup beet juice

½ cup carrot juice

½ cup nettle juice

2–3 tablespoons lemon or lime juice

Mix together the beet, carrot, and nettle juice in a pitcher. Stir in the citrus juice and serve.

Nettle Beer

Nettle beer is a delicious traditional country drink that relieves gout and arthritis. It contains no detectable amount of alcohol and can be enjoyed by those young and old. You'll need 10 (12-ounce) sterilized bottles with corks.

Makes 1 gallon

1 gallon spring water

4 cups young nettle tops

1 tablespoon chopped fresh ginger

1 unpeeled lemon, chopped

2 packed cups brown sugar

4 tablespoons cream of tartar

4½ teaspoons active fresh yeast

1 teaspoon brewer's yeast powder

1. Combine the water, nettles, and ginger in a large pot over medium-high heat. Cook at a low boil, with the lid on, for 15 minutes.

2. Strain the liquid through a fine-mesh strainer or several layers of cheese-cloth into a bowl (discard the solids). Add the lemon, sugar, and cream of tartar. Stir well and let cool to room temperature.

3. Add the yeasts. Cover the bowl with a cloth and keep it on a counter at room temperature for 3 days. Strain into bottles and cork.

4. Let sit at room temperature in a cool, dark place for 1 to 2 weeks before drinking. Store unused portions in the refrigerator.

Nettle Wine

This recipe is adapted from *Wine from the Wilds* by Steven A. Krause. You'll need a large heatproof crock, a fermentation jug, and cheesecloth in addition to wine yeast.

Makes 1 gallon

16 cups young nettle tops

7 cups sugar

4–5 tablespoons orange juice (from 1 orange)

2–3 tablespoons lemon juice (from 1 lemon)

1 gallon boiling water

1 ounce wine yeast

1. Wearing gloves, bruise the nettles by twisting the stalks. Place the bruised nettles in a large crock with the sugar, orange juice, and lemon juice.

2. Pour the boiling water over the nettle mixture. Let cool to room temperature, and stir in the yeast.

3. Cover the crock with a piece of cheesecloth and allow it to sit on a counter at room temperature for 5 days, stirring once each day. Strain into a fermentation jug and seal. Ferment for 3 months to 1 year, or until aged to your taste.

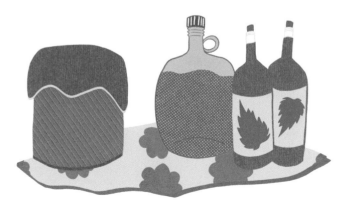

Bibliography

Belaiche, P., and O. Lievoux. "Clinical Studies on the Palliative Treatment of Prostatic Adenoma with Extract of *Urtica* Root." *Phytotherapy Research* 5 (December 1991): 267–69.

Boutenko, Sergei. *Wild Edibles: A Practical Guide to Foraging, with Easy Identification of 60 Edible Plants and 67 Recipes*. Berkeley, CA: North Atlantic Books, 2013.

Brill, "Wildman" Steve, and Evelyn Dean. *Identifying and Harvesting Edible and Medicinal Plants in Wild (and Not So Wild) Places*. New York: HarperCollins, 1994.

Burgess, Isla. *Weeds Heal: A Working Herbal*. Christchurch, NZ: Caxton Press, 1998.

Cech, Richo. *Making Plant Medicine*. Williams, OR: Horizon Herbs Publication, 2000.

Coon, Nelson. *Using Wayside Plants*. New York: Hearthside Press, 1960.

Cox, I. M., et al. "Red Blood Cell Magnesium and Chronic Fatigue Syndrome." *Lancet* 337 (March 30, 1991): 757–60.

Edwards, Gail Faith. *Opening Our Wild Hearts to the Healing Herbs*. Woodstock, NY: Ash Tree Publishing, 2000.

Fischer-Rizzi, Susanne. *Medicine of the Earth: Legends, Recipes, Remedies, and Cultivation of Healing Plants*. Portland, OR: Rudra Press, 1996.

Geelhoed, Glenn W., Robert D. Willix, and Jean Barilla, eds. *Natural Health Secrets from Around the World*. New Canaan, CT: Keats Publishing, 1997.

Hatfield, Audrey Wynne. *Pleasures of Wild Plants*. London: Museum Press Limited, 1966.

Heinerman, John. *Heinerman's Encyclopedia of Healing Juices*. West Nyack, NY: Parker Publishing Company, 1994.

Hitchcock, C. Leo, and Arthur Cronquist. *Flora of the Pacific Northwest: An Illustrated Manual*. Seattle: University of Washington Press, 1973.

Holmes, Peter. *The Energetics of Western Herbs: An Herbal Reference Integrating Western and Oriental Herbal Medicine Traditions*. Boulder, CO: Artemis Press, 1989.

Jones, Pamela. *Just Weeds: History, Myths, and Uses*. New York: Prentice Hall Press, 1991.

Kirk, Donald R. *Wild Edible Plants of Western North America*. Happy Camp, CA: Naturegraph Publishing, 1975.

Mars, Brigitte. *The Desktop Guide to Herbal Medicine*. Laguna Beach, CA: Basic Health Publications, 2016.

Martin, Laura C. *Wildflower Folklore*. Old Saybrook, CT: Globe Pequot Press, 1993.

McIntyre, Anne. *Flower Power: Flower Remedies for Healing Body and Soul through Herbalism, Homeopathy, Aromatherapy, and Flower Essences*. New York: Henry Holt and Company, 1996.

Mills, Simon Y. *The Essential Book of Herbal Medicine*. London: Penguin Arkana, 1994.

Mittman, P. "Randomized, Double-Blind Study of Freeze-Dried *Urtica dioica* in the Treatment of Allergic Rhinitis." *Planta Medica* 56 (February 1990): 44–47.

Onstad, Dianne. *Whole Foods Companion: A Guide for Adventurous Cooks, Curious Shoppers, and Lovers of Natural Foods*. White River Junction, VT: Chelsea Green Publishing, 1996.

Pedersen, Mark. *Nutritional Herbology: A Reference Guide to Herbs*. Warsaw, IN: Wendell Whitman Company, 1995.

Pfeiffer, Ehrenfried. *Weeds and What They Tell Us*. Wyoming, RI: Bio-Dynamic Literature, 1981.

Rogers, Robert Dale. *Rogers' Herbal Manual*. Edmonton, AB: Karamat Wilderness Ways, 2000.

Rothkranz, Markus. *Free Food and Medicine: Worldwide Edible Plant Guide*. Rothkranz Publishing, 2012.

Rutherford, Meg. *A Pattern of Herbs: Herbs for Goodness, Food, and Health and How to Identify and Grow Them*. Garden City, NY: Doubleday Dolphin Book, 1975.

Schofield, Janice J. *Discovering Wild Plants: Alaska, Western Canada, the Northwest*. Anchorage: Alaska Northwest Books, 1989.

Skenderi, Gazmend. *Herbal Vade Mecum*. Rutherford, NJ: Herbacy Press, 2004.

Thayer, Samuel. *The Forager's Harvest: A Guide to Identifying, Harvesting, and Preparing Edible Wild Plants*. Ogema, WI: Forager's Harvest Press, 2006.

Tilford, Gregory. *Edible and Medicinal Plants of the West*. Missoula, MT: Mountain Press, 1997.

Weed, Susun S. *Healing Wise*. Woodstock, NY: Ash Tree Publishing, 1989.

———. *Menopausal Years*. Woodstock, NY: Ash Tree Publishing, 1992.

Westrich, LoLo. *California Herbal Remedies: The History and Uses of Native Medicinal Plants*. Houston: Gulf Publishing, 1989.

Wood, Matthew. *The Earthwise Herbal, Volume I: A Complete Guide to Old World Medicinal Plants*. Berkeley, CA: North Atlantic Books, 2008.

Resources

NETTLE SEEDS
Strictly Medicinal Seeds, LLC
https://strictlymedicinalseeds.com

MAIL ORDER NETTLES AND NETTLE PRODUCTS
Rebecca's Herbal Apothecary
https://rebeccasherbs.com

JUST FOR FUN
Here is a song about nettles by my partner, BethyLoveLight, that also shows the nettle patch next to our home!
https://www.youtube.com/watch?v=ULDI7XkLBbs

Metric Conversion Charts

Weight

TO CONVERT	TO	MULTIPLY
ounces	grams	ounces by 28.35
pounds	grams	pounds by 453.5
pounds	kilograms	pounds by 0.45

Volume

TO CONVERT	TO	MULTIPLY
teaspoons	milliliters	teaspoons by 4.93
tablespoons	milliliters	tablespoons by 14.79
fluid ounces	milliliters	fluid ounces by 29.57
cups	milliliters	cups by 236.59
cups	liters	cups by 0.24
pints	milliliters	pints by 473.18
pints	liters	pints by 0.473
quarts	milliliters	quarts by 946.36
quarts	liters	quarts by 0.946
gallons	liters	gallons by 3.785

Index

Page numbers in *italics* indicate illustrations; numbers in **bold** indicate charts.